Simpson Protocol

From the Inside

Case studies, Insights and Observations from the People who use the Simpson Protocol Process on a daily basis.

A look at one of the most advanced and up to date methods for using Hypnosis as Therapy in the world today.

Winner of the **'Hypnosis Pioneer Award" 2014**

Complied by Ines Simpson

SIMPSON PROTOCOL from the Inside

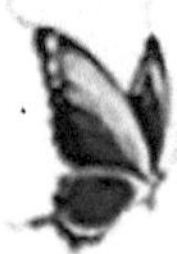

Copyright ©
2024
Ines Simpson

All rights reserved. No part of this publication may be reproduced, stored in a retrieval system, or transmitted in any form or by any means, electronic, mechanical, photocopying, recording, or otherwise, without the prior written permission of the copyright holder.

ISBN 978-1-0690045-1-2

An InesSimpson Press Publication

Ines Simpson
www.inessimpsonhypnosis.com

Further Info: https://simpsonprotocol.com/

Personal Stories and I Case Studies from SP Practitioners who are creating and expanding the world of Simpson Protocol.

Explore the transformative world of Simpson Protocol (SP) through the eyes of practitioners who are pushing the boundaries of what's possible with this process.

In this compelling collection of personal stories and real-life case studies, you'll discover how SP has become a catalyst for profound change—whether physical, mental, emotional, or spiritual.

Through these pages, you'll witness sessions that often seem nothing short of miraculous, addressing and neutralizing the deepest traumas to create lasting positive outcomes. From the simple to the complex, there is no human issue beyond the reach of Simpson Protocol, as it taps into the limitless potential of the client's higher mind.

Whether you're a seasoned practitioner or new to the world of hypnosis as therapy, this book offers invaluable insights and inspiration. Read on to discover how SP is changing lives—and how it might change yours.

Contents

List of Contributors

Andreas Bacher

Angela Freychet

Annamaria LaScala

Birgit Alaya Brinkpeter

Christophe Dierckx

Claudia Dagnino

Corrie van Pinxteren

Deepali Agarwal

Fay Kelly

Greg Beckett

Hana Zawodny

Hanne Essers

Heidi Puffing

Helene Sousa

Honey Lansdowne

Imane Soubra

Isi Murray

Justine Lette

Liesbeth Meuldijk

Lily McKenzie

Ludovic Louissaint

Manuela Rauch

Marianne Eelen

Michael Stier

Miranda Geens

Nancy Schilder

Nicole Ah-Von

Patricia (Patty) Meier

Paul Arnaud

Phil Cardow

Rachael Hay

Sandra Schaighofer

Stin-Niels Musche

Tanja Eich

Tim Horn

William Salama

Yasmin Udwadia

Zhi Yang

Introduction

With this book you will have an inside look at one of the most advanced and up to date methods for using Modern Hypnosis as Therapy in the world today.

Now the first thing to know about the Simpson Protocol (SP) process is – it's never finished. It's not fixed – it's always evolving.

It's evolving because we are constantly finding new needs it can meet and because individual practitioners bring new insights to the process.

In this Book you will see, some of the different viewpoints, and different ways SP is used by these SP practitioners around the world.

The second thing to know is – this is not exclusively for Hypnotists – it's for anyone looking for the most comprehensive (we say, Holistic) way to use self-care for patients, clients, friends, family and themselves.

What is this Book about?

This is a look at SP (Simpson Protocol) from the inside, stories case studies, and client testimonials all involving the SP process, and the results and outcomes from the process.

When you use SP Self Hypnosis – you also have the most complete Self-Help tool you could find.

SP can be the one stop shop tool for any and every issue and issues you encounter as a Professional Therapist. As Ines Simpson always says when her students ask her – "What does SP do best?"

 "Everything!!"

Inside this book, on these pages you will find a wide variety of viewpoints on SP, its methods, and what it can achieve. It is the most comprehensive record we have to date – across all types, all professions and all languages.

We created this book from all the articles and case studies that were sent in by Practicing SP practitioners.

And I have added some bits and pieces to take a reader on the journey and evolution of SP.

At the end of the book is a little history about how SP evolved.

How to read this book

Of course, you can read the same way you read any other book – just start at the beginning and keep going till it's all done!

Or if you are a Practitioner, perhaps you want to jump to some of the case studies – listed in the contents.

Or if you are brand new to the concept of Hypnosis as therapy but have picked this book up out of curiosity – perhaps you may want to look at the sections where I describe and explain various attributes of the SP Process – just go anything headed 'NOTE' – where I point out many of the unique and interesting aspects of this process.

And this book will also take you along on the Journey of SP as it grew and developed into a worldwide process.

At the end of the book, I talk about the Simpson Protocol, what it can do and why.

Or, of course, feel free to just flip through the book – everyone has a story to tell, and they all have their own flavor.

Please enjoy.

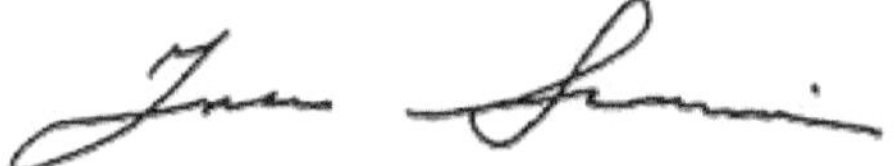

Some Explanations for words and concepts used by the Contributors.

Peace, Deep, High: These are 'trigger words' that are set in the first session you have with an SP Practitioner. They allow you to go into a nice state of trance anytime – just by saying them or intending them. So, you can use SP Self Hypnosis anytime. Also, when you go back (if you need) for a second or subsequent SP session – there are no more inductions. You say or intend the trigger words, and you get right to work.

SuperConscious: The driver of the Simpson Protocol process. At first SP was a process that allowed a practitioner to use the deep Esdaile state to work with a Client. Gradually SP became the connection of the Practitioner and the Client to this thing we call the SuperConscious. The energy and wisdom that does all the work in the session and creates the great outcomes we witness using SP. There is more on the SuperConscious at the end of the book.

Divine: A code word for a place or a state where the Client can connect directly with the Universe, the Source – something amazing. And each experience is deeply felt and personal to each Client.

Entities: 'Entities' in Hypnosis mean an energy apart from the Client's core being. Can be positive or negative. Can be suppressed emotions, can be outside energies. It's a wide term.

Multiple Souls: We have discovered in our journey with SP, that a person can have more than one Soul. Usually, they are there to help or learn. But sometimes they need to leave or start to hinder the person's journey. All can be investigated with SP.

Surrogate Hypnosis: This is where 'a surrogate' stands in for the Client. Typically, a family member. A mother enters Hypnosis to allow work on her child. Or a person is in a coma and a family member would like to connect. It's also known to have a great effect on animals. Where an owner can be connected to their animal and heal any upsets the animal is encountering.

In Surrogate Hypnosis: Both parties connect at the highest level (with permission) – there is no conscious connection.

Chapter 1- SP Getting Started

NOTE: Ines Simpson

I developed over time this process that became known as Simpson Protocol.

I had learnt the core of my Hypnosis training from Jerry Kein. Jerry Kein, one of the outstanding figures in Modern Hypnosis, was an amazing teacher and mentor for me, teaching me to appreciate the art and science of Hypnosis.

Jerry Kein at that time was a presenter at NGH (National Guild of Hypnotists) Conventions that I attended annually.

And as I gained Confidence, I began to teach at the NGH.

At first, I taught a process called 'Working in Esdaile and Beyond.' How to set your Client up to communicate in the Esdaile state – this gradually morphed into a version of SP.

I was joined by Ted Robinson for a while – an expert in EFT (Emotional Freedom Technique) and we taught our classes together. Ted helped me immensely to get SP established in those early days.

I think the first SP Class I ever did was in Seattle, Washington- set up by Ray Zukowski

However, it really took off when, at one of those NGH presentations, a certain, Stin-Neils Musche was in the audience. As were a couple of gentlemen called Hansruedi Wipf, Hanspeter Ricklin who invited me to a Hypnosis Convention they were creating in Zurich Switzerland.

SP was going international!

But it was the connection I had with Stin-Niels Musche that made SP truly expand its reach.

Consider the first training he set up for me in Germany had about 25 attendees – which was amazing for a teacher no one had ever heard of, and a process no-one had ever heard of!

SP is now a Worldwide process – but it was Germany where we started to really create traction for SP – so let's start this journey in Germany.

And I will be back to jump in throughout the book.

GERMANY and AUSTRIA

Stin-Niels Musche, SP Trainer Germany

When I first met Ms. Simpson, I had walked into a convention hall wearing a baseball cap, Ms. Simpson spotted me and exclaimed, 'Hey, there's my Facebook friend!' It was surprising because I looked nothing like my Facebook profile.

And later, at the Convention Diner and Dance, we danced together, of all things! But it was fun and that was the beginning of an amazing connection that has lasted ever since.

I began my career as an insurance broker in Germany, eventually transitioning into sales and communication training. Then, unexpectedly, hypnosis crossed my path. I stumbled upon the great Hypnotist, Jerry Kein, who happened to be Ines's mentor as well. From Jerry, I learned hypnosis with a focus on Regression Therapy.

I never delved into Ericksonian style or other hypnosis approaches because I found regression therapy incredibly effective. Despite its challenges, I still enjoy using it occasionally, even though I know some may find it easier to use different methods.

Still, I sought something more efficient than regression therapy. I desired a holistic approach that felt lighter for both clients and me. That's when I heard about the Simpson Protocol. It was thought to be unconventional – but I found it intriguing. However, at that time, it was hard to get any real information, as Ms. Simpson didn't have much about it on the Internet at that time.

But, when I witnessed her demonstration of the process at a convention, I was captivated.

It felt like discovering the Holy Grail of hypnosis—a holistic, emotionally gentle approach that promised better outcomes for clients.

 That was about ten years ago, and ever since that day, I've been in love with the Simpson Protocol, and over those years I have watched it develop so much further – allowing its Practitioners to do so much more.

In the early days, mastering Simpson Protocol was challenging, especially with each session being unique, and based on the client's needs. The structure was there, but it was difficult to grasp fully. I bought the DVDs and watched demos repeatedly, trying to decipher the process and jotting down what I understood.

Ms. Simpson did every demo differently it seemed to me – because each demo she did was catering to the Client she was working on, not the students who were trying to learn. Which is a good thing for the Client – but it wasn't easy for me to learn.

However, what kept me coming back was the ease and effectiveness of the process, especially how she used regression within Simpson Protocol. As I persisted, attending classes, and watching Ines teach, the method began to make sense.

As I said Ms. Simpson and I had formed a strong connection, and I was wondering if she would consider letting me teach Simpson Protocol in Germany. Before I could reach out, she contacted me and offered me the opportunity to become the SP trainer in Germany. I eagerly accepted.

My goal, even back then, was to make SP the Gold Standard for Hypnosis in Germany. And I do believe we have succeeded in that goal.

I've witnessed the Simpson Protocol evolve over time, always moving towards being more inclusive, able to take on more and more issues and at the same paring down the process to make it simpler – both for the Client and the Practitioner.

'Less creates More' is the philosophy of SP.

And it's in continual development, aiming for better outcomes for clients and making the process smoother for hypnotists. I truly appreciate that aspect of it—it's always evolving and improving.

And to the question who can benefit from the SP Process?

Every individual dealing with people from various aspects of health—not just emotional health—can benefit. I often encounter patients with physical ailments seeking assistance, and we're able to improve their outcomes. Additionally, nowadays, I see clients struggling with financial or success-related beliefs affecting their jobs. Essentially, any issue connected to the mind can be addressed and aided.

Stin-Niels Musche   stin-niels.musche@gmx.de

INES SIMPSON an aside

The first trainings we did together in Germany – in wonderful Potsdam – were 'interesting.'

Stin would translate – so I would say a sentence and then wait while the sentence became a paragraph (it seemed) in German.

Of course, I would often forget to stop to allow him to translate - then I would hear "Ms. Simpson, Ms. Simpson – Stop! Stop! – my turn"!

Stin and his partner Martin eventually moved to Hamburg, where Stin set up HypnoSchool and continued to advance the awareness throughout the whole of the German speaking world.

However, I loved Potsdam, and really enjoyed the visits to Sanssouci. My first taste of Germany!

Insights and observations from some German Practitioners

Andreas Bacher, SP Practitioner

Austria

After a hypnosis training in 2019 with a German colleague and during a further training with the Yager Code I became aware of the Simpson Protocol.

I took the training and since then I have been working with my clients exclusively with the SP, because that's where I have the most success.

Case Study

I worked with a young man who had major self-esteem issues and as a result no longer felt comfortable in his body. He also had problems at school as he suffered from test anxiety and learning blocks.

After consulting with his mother and himself, we agreed on 3 sessions with an interval of about 5 weeks.

Even after the first session, the 15-year-old's mother told me that there had been huge improvements in his behavior.

After successfully completing all the sessions, I was informed that he had become a model pupil at school, as his whole behavior and nature had changed. And he now genuinely enjoys all aspects of learning.

His mother is infinitely grateful for this change in behavior and the young man is also happy that he chose and took this step.

Andreas Bacher mindpower4you.AB@gmail.com

Michael Stier, SP Practitioner

Germany

My background lies in the world of insurance and the study of criminology and criminal law. My focus was on white-collar crime. However, in 2015, I realized that this wasn't my life's path. Without knowing what would come next, I left the company. Delving into complex processes had always been my talent.

My journey began when my wife underwent hypnosis. That was my first exposure to this world, and I was amazed at how quickly psychological issues could be resolved. Initially, I learned about regression hypnosis and the Yager Code. But my curiosity led me to the Simpson Protocol, not merely a technique but a process. Today, I specialize in external energies, souls, spirits, and demons.

My Own Case Study

It was 2020 when a client with anxieties and constant pressure in her throat came to me. She constantly spat mucus. Foreign energy blocked any access to her. After removing the blockages, I successfully worked with the Simpson Protocol. Proudly, I went to bed exhausted in the evening, needing rest. I woke up at 4 am, immediately aware that I had absorbed this foreign energy, which I then sent away. After a week, my wife felt weak, with throat complaints. When she told me, I knew where that energy had gone, from me to my wife. That wasn't funny.

I learned that just sending foreign energy into the light wasn't enough. I began furthering my education in the field of foreign energies, spirits, and demons from mentors in the USA, Poland, and Switzerland.

An interesting event from 2023:

A young nurse came to me, accompanied by her mother. Initially, she wanted to turn back at the door, fearing what might happen in the hypnosis session. Panic attacks plagued her, mainly on her way to work. She loved her job but couldn't understand why these panic attacks occurred.

In the preliminary discussion, I reassured her and began trance induction. She quickly fell into a panic attack, which I immediately recognized due to my sensitivity to foreign energies and sent her into the light. But they returned in the evening, stronger than before. I was aware and had warned the client.

In the second session, I managed to telepathically communicate with the foreign energy, revealing a deceased woman from the hospital. She had experienced great pain in the hospital and, after her death, clung to the nurse there, living off her life energy. This explained the panic attacks on the way to work, as the deceased soul naturally didn't want to return to the place of her painful experiences and death.

I had to gently explain to the client that a foreign soul was occupying her. Not easy when the client has no reference to such matters. Due to constant overtime, she was physically and mentally weakened, making her vulnerable and allowing entry to such energies. Alcohol, drugs, illness, and excessive work can cause our protective aura to be compromised.

The process of leading such souls into the light requires trust and sensitivity. Communication in the Simpson Protocol through finger signals allowed me to exchange with the foreign soul. I asked her if she loved her parents, and she said no because she was raised by her grandparents. I asked if it would be okay to call the souls of her grandparents, to which she agreed.

After clarifying conversations with the soul's grandparents, I managed to convey what awaited her in the light of God. She agreed to go with them as companions and be guided into the light. This is not a Hollywood exorcism story but hard work.

To all readers, caution is advised: Avoid trying magical games like Ouija boards for fun or delving into dark magic or voodoo, summoning spirits of the deceased without understanding it. Everything has its price.

Here is my Opinion and my Opinion only from my Experiences with this kind of work:

Therapeutic work with external energies usually requires 1-3 months of work and the client's willingness to let go of the foreign energy. Some clients identify so strongly with this foreign energy that sometimes no healing is possible. I think of the realm of schizophrenia or even borderline personality disorder. Our psychiatric facilities are full of spiritually occupied people.

As long as a person's free will is strong, therapeutic help can be given.

The nurse now lives without fear and panic with her family. Through the Simpson Protocol, I, as a therapist, can communicate with these energies through finger signals. It's an excellent tool to be a translator between worlds.

Michael Stier stiermi@me.com

Heidi Puffing, SP Practitioner

Graz, Austria

I worked as a qualified nurse for 15 years and was also involved in clinical research. My vitae also include a university degree in case and care management. I have been self-employed for four years and work full-time as a qualified hypnotist.

Two years ago, I came across the Simpson Protocol on the Internet and was immediately fascinated. After finding a colleague who used the Simpson Protocol Process, I booked my first session and asked numerous questions about it. The experience during the session and, above all, the results achieved convinced me that I wanted to offer this method to my own clients. Two months later, I decided to train in the Simpson Protocol Process and become a Simpson Protocol Practitioner.

I have been using the Simpson Protocol in my practice for almost two years now, having worked as a hypnotist for four years. However, the effects that I have observed in both my clients and I from using the SP have often left me speechless. Particularly impressive was the depth and range of the results achieved.

A Case Study

One of my first clients to use the Simpson Protocol was a 67-year-old lady who suffered from massive insomnia that had been going on for seven years and was already having a significant impact on her.

She had already tried numerous methods and medications, including an unsuccessful attempt at classical hypnosis. After using SP, she was not only able to sleep 6-7 hours a night again after seven years, but also reported that for the first time in her life she stood up for herself, suddenly set boundaries and said "no", which she had not been able to do before. As a result, she had experienced her world in a new way and had, among other things, gained far more peace and serenity. These changes were lasting and are still there today, as she recently told me.

I am always impressed by how the Superconscious mind takes care of all the underlying issues without me as a hypnotherapist needing to know anything about them. I only found out about some of the issues that affected clients but which they hadn't mentioned (which isn't necessary with SP) through their reviews and feedback. I would like to share one client's Google feedback here in her own words. In the first session, the client had only mentioned that she felt unhappy and had little interest in anything anymore:

Mrs. A. 28 years old, tells:

I'm finally living instead of just functioning.

I am an atheist and a rather skeptical person who is not completely closed to new experiences.

I went to Heidi with the attitude: "Yes, it can work, but it doesn't have to" and with a lot of baggage.

Having suffered from years of recurring depressive moods, anxiety, panic attacks and unresolved conflicts from childhood, I had already been to therapy and tried various methods to grow and to be able to live/enjoy/live my life, at least in the meantime.

I learned a lot and was given many useful tools to somehow manage my life. Sometimes better, sometimes worse.

But it was never easy and there was always the fear that the next down would drag me down. Hopefully not too deep, hopefully not too long, hopefully I wouldn't lose too much... No matter how well I had the tools under control in between, it was never natural, never easy, never automatic like breathing.

I had already resigned myself to having to go to therapy for the rest of my life so that I could somehow function. From today's perspective, it sounds sadder than it was back then. I didn't know anything else, the longing for "different" was never great because I couldn't imagine "different".

I then became aware of Heidi through friends and acquaintances. I watched it from the sidelines for two years. "What if it helps, but then I'm no longer me?"

 "Who am I anyway, and do I even want to be someone else just so that I feel "better?"

My fears, my insecurities, my impulsiveness, my imbalances had become a huge part of my personality, what would be left if I "lost" it all? What if I was "wiped out" and someone else was left?

Through a very heavy blow of fate, I then decided enough is enough. And the worst thing that could happen? I either got better or nothing happened - because there was no worse.

The first thing I can say about SP Hypnosis is that it is different from what most people probably imagine. There are different types of hypnosis - most famously "I count to three and you're a chicken..."

I did a different kind of hypnosis with Heidi, where I was always "there" and yet knew from about halfway through that this is trance, this is hypnosis.

Heidi gave me the tools to work with myself, anytime and anywhere. Since I've had these tools (Self- hypnosis), I can actually reduce my stress to Zero.

Again, my fears and insecurities are bit there in between and okay, but no longer overwhelming and above all they no longer possess me.

I am still me, but I have a life that I can finally enjoy. I can finally look forward to tomorrow/cinema/dinner/sitting with friends/etc. again without lying or pretending.

It's no longer an endless loop of task I have to work through to make it seem like I'm living.

I know Heidi, you'll say now that you were "just guiding" and that I deserve all this work and praise myself. But I could never have done it all without you.

Thank you so much for giving me my life back." A.

Once again, I witnessed how the Simpson Protocol and Superconsciousness works in a wonderful way, as it has done so many times before. In the meantime, this client has also been able to completely overcome her remaining fears and insecurities. I am extremely grateful to have the Simpson Protocol as a tool with which I have already been able to successfully help many people to improve their quality of life and overcome stressful issues.

Heidi Puffing   info@hypnose-vida.at

Ines Simpson- SP for Clearing spaces

From an email Heidi sent to me

What I have wanted to ask you for a long time, have you ever worked with the superconscious on cleaning space and property? I tried it relatively early on in my SP work and played with it and was thrilled beyond words. I know it from Reiki but with Reiki it takes a long time, and it is not possible to "download" specific energies into certain areas.

For example, in my practice I asked SC to first cleanse the rooms and the property energetically, to clear low vibrational energies, to remove all blockages that could interfere with my work, etc.

Then I went into detail: when the clients walk through the door, they feel relax and feel comfortable, the corresponding energy/frequency in the chair where they are sitting- speak freely about their topic, in the hypnosis chair easily, simply go into a trance etc., my chair is surrounded by a protection and energy of concentration, my intuition is strengthened etc. It has more than exceeded my expectations!!!

I had to change the thing with client speaking free, because they no longer stopped talking.

From then on, I always heard from clients who came in "the room is so incredibly bright and beautiful", and I also noticed how comfortable and relaxed they felt, and clients went into a trance incredibly quickly.

I expanded it and first tested it in my apartment...something like the energy at the bedroom door, that relaxation and calmness sets in when I walk through, the energy/frequency for a restful, regenerative healthy sleep etc. over the bed. Since it worked so wonderfully, I also used it with clients. When I had a client with sleep problems, I added it to the classic SP session. A mom once told me her 4-year-old son always comes to her bed at night and she doesn't sleep well, so I did this in his room and since then he has stayed in his room every night (except when he was ill). I also add it to weight loss topics, in the kitchen I intuitively use the energy to eat healthy food that helps with weight loss for this person, creativity, healthy balanced cooking, etc.

Now when I was sick with Covid, I asked SC (in addition to the health program) to add the energy for physical healing and the frequencies of the color that serves healing above my bed for this time - I was by the way healthy within 4 days.

When I first did it, I just wrote everything on paper and asked SC if it can do it worked perfectly.

Heidi Puffing

Manuela Rauch, SP Practitioner

Austria

A Session

When Client A was with me last week, we had a really great session. When I asked the basics, it went very well, although there was something there with external energy, but it could be sent away without further ado. And then we were able to work really well on her issue, it didn't even block, just great. When we finished the session, she was beaming all over her face. Her mother noticed it too and called me later.

"Something has changed for me too, since I had the session with you, there was something else with external energies, but this time I dealt with it differently. I also asked if we needed to go to another level so that we could send this entity away, and the yes finger came. And it could then be sent away as normal. I have the feeling that I am no longer so afraid of it and can accept it better. Last week I didn't have a difficult external energy, which for me is a sign that I have learned."

Since I've been working with the SP program, it's been leading me to such tasks again and again and if I don't get it, then the topic comes up until I've learned it. I once had a client who had no less than 10 causes and experiences that she wanted to look at with her Experiences that it wanted to look at with consciousness. I have never had so many in one session.

With the six positive experiences, I thought to myself that the client was too conscious. I couldn't understand why only positive situations came up, then I had a thought and asked the superconscious whether a resource should be taken from this situation that was brought to a positive 10. Then a yes came and I anchored this resource so that the feeling comes up whenever she needs it without needing an impulse from her. And lo and behold, the negative experience came up for me to work on. I think it's just fantastic how the Superconscious guides you, even if I don't always understand it at first go

In another session I had a little boy, Björn is 6 years old and came because he couldn't concentrate so well, but also because he had a lot of anger in him.

Björn came to me and told me that he was happy that I was helping him to get rid of this anger. What was interesting about him was that I didn't feel like I was talking to a 6-year-old, but to someone who knows how to work with the Superconscious. He said during the session that he had two souls, and one was holding on to the anger and he didn't want this anger.

And at the end when the concentration waned, and I thought I could ask two more questions. He said that he was coming back now and could therefore no longer answer my questions from within, that he no longer had access to them. At the second session he asked me if he could also ask my Superconscious a question. I asked what he wanted to know. He said how old my soul really is.

I then said, do you mean my age? He said no, that of your soul. That was two really strange sessions.

In a session with Client Ms. XY, it was the 3rd session on the topic of letting go of the past. When I wanted to end the session, the no finger came, I queried pretty much everything and was at a loss as to why the Superconscious wouldn't let me finish. Then I asked if the Superconscious mind could send clear information to Mrs. XY in the form of thoughts; Pictures, feelings, why I am not allowed to finish this session yet. Mrs. XY then said cigarettes, she saw cigarettes.

I then got her out of hypnosis and asked her if she would be willing to let her cigarettes go?

 Yes, she would be willing to do so. When she was at High again, we

did this non-smoking hypnosis in about 15 minutes. She is still a non-smoker today and has never had any needs or thoughts about smoking. These are great experiences if you get involved in them.

Manuela Rauch   hypnose-bei-manuela.com

Tanja Eich, SP Practitioner

Germany

I only did the training in March 2023 and have already experienced some positive things:

1. I did Surrogate hypnosis for my daughter during the seminar - no specific topic - a few days later she contacted me and reported that she went to work, got into the elevator to the office - and only in the elevator did she realize she was in it. She had always avoided it because of her fear of elevators. On this day, she used the elevator without thinking.

2) A client with hypochondriacal traits - she is a doctor herself - had success in the first session in that she can now read articles about cancer in a completely neutral way without thinking that she would now develop it herself. (She had cancer at a young age)

3. A client went to the toilet after the session and came back and told me that she had just not recognized herself in the mirror because

such a positive face was looking back at her. A few weeks later, this client went on a long car journey all by herself - without first considering whether she had the confidence to do so.

4) A client came to me because she was very anxious about invasive procedures. However, her superconscious wanted to work on a different issue. As a result, she has now started to tidy up her life. She tells me that she has put the images she saw while solving the questions into practice at home. She has also been approached by other people about how positive she looks on the outside, which is also noticeable on her face.

5. When I asked a client at the end of the session to classify the feeling about her issue on a scale of 1-10, she was totally

overwhelmed that the feeling was only at 2, it had always been at least 12 before!

These are just a few experiences I can share - I'm sure there will be MANY more!

Tanja Eich www.tanjaeich.de

Ines Simpson *Now two amazing women, who I am privileged to know personally – who do amazing work.*

Sandra Schwaighofer and Birgit Alaya Brinkpeter.

Sandra Schwaighofer, SP Practitioner

Austria

If our feelings meet our thoughts, we create our reality. How SP transformed my life unexpectedly.

As a Certified. SP Practitioner, hypnotherapist, mind coach (and former opera singer) human beings have always been the key point of my interest: People - "being human in itself" are my great passion.

Hypnosis united the different fields of my education, my interests and my profession: hypnotherapy, mind training and theatre/music/art. In all three fields I have been using hypnosis ever since, even if I had not been consciously aware of it at the beginning. And at a certain point in time, it also changed my life profoundly. On all levels of my conscious and non-conscious mind.

What is it that must be healed, to call us "Healthy "?

Personal crisis

In 2016 a severe infection in my right eye caused by acanthamoeba threatened my health and I became heavily sick for many years.

In one day, I was torn out of my beloved job at the theatre, torn out of my family life, torn out of my social life. And suddenly instead of being a happy high achiever, a mother of two beloved children and a happy wife, my soul was slowly dying, murdered by ruthless parasites, and a tortured body that was slowly being eaten by living creatures I could not see, but which caused excruciating pain.

The treatment resembled further torture: irregular sleep for years (because I needed a certain medicine every 1– 2 hours/24h a day), terrible chronic pain, living in total darkness for over a year. Regular operations (nearly 20 over 4 years), lying for weeks either only on my stomach or (depending on the medical issue) on my back. Cruel medical procedures. Not able to see, not able to move my eyeballs, stuck in an almost hopeless situation. Doctors that could not help me or had been too late to help me successfully.

Eventually it was all over. But after three years of waiting for my health to restore my job at the theatre was gone; in the fourth year my marriage was broken; in the fifth year both children were damaged by the subsequent traumatic separation and splitting through certain family members. Plus, through that whole time my father was slowly dying of cancer at home. My whole world had been turned upside down. My world had been shattered into a thousand pieces.

As a consequence, I started to suffer from severe PTSD. I was emotionally, physically, mentally and spiritually broken, a shadow of my former self. (And I had been a radiant, shining, strong person with high spirits before all that).

Through the medical treatment I was physically burned out, abandoned by what I thought had been my friends, trampled over by abusive people, who I had thought would love and support me in these difficult times.

But I knew that giving up was not an option. That I literally had to look my greatest fears, my greatest sorrows, into the eye. And that I had to help myself, because nobody else would do it. That suicide was no option. Because I knew that though this inner light that had used to shine within me, that seemed lost now – that this light was still there, somewhere deep inside me.

Searching the Internet for answers, for help, for anything – I stumbled across information about Simpson Protocol.

After my first session – an SP Self-Hypnosis session - my PTSD was totally gone!

This was the turning point in my life.

And I thought, if this first 'test' session could create this change in me – and at that time, after all I had been through – it felt like a miracle – what could this 'miracle' of SP do for others?

And since that time, as I built up my client base again - this miracle has been also allowed to happen over and over again for my clients.

Also, many personal sessions would follow after that, because I finally was ready to really allow healing to myself from my inner core. This was a huge shift in my life. It was like a huge transformational process, where I finally could build up my whole personality, my whole existence anew. It felt like coming home after a long, long dark journey. It saved my life. And it opened me up to all possibilities – even the first seemingly impossible ones.

Since then, I was able to return to my professional life again. Found my new second dream job as a hypnotherapist and mind trainer. Found new friends, a new life, new happiness and joy.

Last but not least: found my inner light again. I could return to my old power, strength and commitment.

SP as the golden key to healing

So, wherever you come from - I feel you. And I want to encourage you: it's worth it!

 Whatever your goal you want to achieve: Go for it!

It's possible, even if it seems impossible at first.

Hypnosis is one of those "tools of mind" that changes lives. Not only mine.

You deserve it as well.

And the Simpson Protocol is one of the *golden keys to healing* on all levels of conscious and non-conscious mind. In our whole system. To the depth of our souls and from the bottom of our hearts.

A sample of Testimonials I have received.

Feedback by a female client Bibiana, Germany: CEO, 43 years

I knew nothing about the Simpson Protocol.

When the corona pandemic was at its peak, my depression slowly but surely lifted its head again and spread through my life. A gray-black heaviness began to take over my everyday life again.

A friend advised me to give the Simpson Protocol a try. So, I contacted Ines Simpson directly, not expecting to receive an answer at all.

But she did! And a few days later we had our first session. I had no great expectations; my biggest worry was falling asleep during the session. I had no idea WHAT to expect during the following hour and how much it would change my life.

But an hour after we started the session, not only was my depression gone, but the leaden blanket that I hadn't even noticed before, because it had been with me for as long as I could remember – was gone.

In the 1950's I read that client, or Volunteers for stage Hypnosis would often sink into a trance state and resist emerging. This we came to find was the Esdaile state, and for the first time these individuals experienced true peace and tranquility in this state. The Hypnotist would have to promise them, they would teach them to go back there on their own – before they would allow themselves to leave that wonderful state.

Consciousness sits in a nice, safe place as you embark on a journey that I would actually describe as a deeply spiritual experience.

Now, one year and three sessions with Ines [Simpson] and four sessions with Sandra Schwaighofer later, things have changed in my life that I never expected.

I have learned to say "no" and set boundaries. I am productive again and can work again.

My writer's block is also gone. What sounds so mundane had an extreme impact on my emotional and professional life.

Writing has always been an expression of my soul. Writing allowed me to entrust my thoughts and worries to paper, to let go.

This outlet was closed to me for years. I couldn't even write new or extra content for my website. So, this writer's block cost me a lot of time and money.

I would never have imagined that you could regain balance and harmony remotely within minutes in a quick hypnosis over the phone in the middle of a café at Edeka! (*German Grocery Store*).

Although... I would say it was so much more.

I can hardly describe in words the impact that these few sessions had on my life, because no problem that we worked on once in a session ever came back. As a scientist might say they balanced my brain chemistry. I only know one thing: it changed my life.

Umar N., Pakistan, student, 19 years old (social anxiety)

Absolutely loved this single session. Learned a lot of new things. I can see many positive changes in myself. I always had a hard time asking questions in class, I was always fearful, but after one session – the fear had gone.

Yasmin N., Dubai: hypnotherapist/mind coach, 55 years

Ms. Schwaighofer is an amazing therapist. I have had a complete life transformation through my sessions with her after a number of extreme experiences throughout my life.

Because of trauma and other experiences – there was a lot I was hoping to resolve. Through the sessions I appreciated the complete privacy of her technique and have been absolutely thrilled by the outstanding outcomes I have achieved after the sessions with her.

As a fellow professional hypnotherapist/mental coach I have learned clinical hypnotherapy and many other formats as well. The Simpson Protocol, that Ms. Schwaighofer is using, I believe, is one of the most advanced and gentlest ways for clients to achieve their goals as fast as possible and resolve deep issues.

The sensitivity, kindness and empathy Mrs. Schwaighofer used to guide me effectively through my sessions with her made me completely trust her abilities and helped me to turn my life around fast in every aspect I turned to her for help. I highly recommend her for any kind of issue. You will be in the best of hands!

Maheen, Pakistan, Software Engineer, 32 years old

Anyone who is feeling lost, suicidal, depressed or anxious. If you are reading this, I would say try this SP Process -because I was one of you.

My words would do no justice to the unbelievably great experience I am having with Sandra's sessions and the Simpson Protocol.

Initially I had doubts about how this process works but at the same time I was open to experiencing it because I was in so much pain that I thought it won't matter even if this therapy doesn't work - I must try.

Before Sandra, I went to two psychologists to fix my issues, but it didn't work, and I was even more suicidal. Sandra has saved not only my life but also, she organized my thoughts and helped me find my life purpose.

The best thing about her SP Process is, she introduced me to the unconditional divine love which we all have in ourselves but it's somehow hidden due to our bad experiences and thought barriers and we crave for this love in others.

I am more at peace and settled within myself, and the world, than ever before.

Thank you so much Sandra for the gems you have taken out and polished them for me. You allowed me to find my life again. A life I had lost forever.

Sandra Schwaighofer simpsonprotocol@gmx.at

Birgit Alaya Brinkpeter, SP Practitioner

Germany

In 2019, after my training with Ines Simpson, I embarked on a transformative journey with the Simpson Protocol that led me to an extraordinary dialogue with the Superconscious Mind. This profound experience unveiled insights that transcend ordinary understanding, revealing the essence of our interconnectedness.

This knowledge is a call to action, a directive to use this understanding to bring about positive change, and to enlighten both ourselves and the world around us.

Here is an excerpt from the dialogue:

"Superconscious Mind" is the part that connects us all. All is one and we are all. You can't define it without limiting it. I am the connection between ALL THAT IS. I am LOVE without words. I am the love of God that connects you. The eternal connection. The connection to all knowledge. I am not a person. I am the love that expresses itself through me, that is formed through me, that is visible through me and finds its expression in everything. You only must look. Through me everything is connected to each other. I am the connection. The connection to the higher realms, to everything, to God. I am the star that sparkles in the sky. The light in the darkness. The light that illuminates the darkness. I am the beauty in every moment. I am the light that unites everything, the connection. The divine spark in everything. The truth. I am infinite in strength and power. Use me only for good. I am life force. The breath of God that animates all. I am You and through You I flow into the world to touch and heal everything and illuminate everything. "

With unwavering love and gratitude Birgit Alaya Brinkpeter

Having experienced various hypnosis styles and learned from multiple teachers, I consider the Simpson Protocol as the missing piece of the puzzle and the connection to All That Is. SP's unique approach, which empowers clients to connect with their own subconscious minds, aligns perfectly with my philosophy of healing from within.

I recognized the profound impact that SP can have on my clients' lives.

Case study:

Meet Sarah, a young and talented female singer whose life was marred by a recurring pattern of disappointment in relationships. She seemed to attract the wrong men, leaving her heartbroken time and again. After a transformative Simpson Protocol session, Sarah experienced a profound shift in her mindset, shifting her focus from seeking external love to true self-love.

This profound shift in resonance transformed her energy and outlook on life, ultimately drawing a man who not only loved her but also resonated with the newfound love she had discovered within.

As within, so without – Sarah shortly after the session drew in a man who had also discovered love for himself. Their connection flourished because he was capable of giving genuine love, having learned to love and value himself.

Together, they exemplified the profound truth that attracting love from others begins with the love we cultivate within ourselves.

The change in Sarah`s heart and the newfound clarity and self-worth became the catalyst for a love story with her soulmate that blossomed into a joyful marriage that changed her life forever. Simpson Protocol unlocked the doors to love and happiness she had been searching for all along.

"These are the miracles of life I am doing my work for, and they are always filling me with deep gratitude."

Testimonials For Birgit

Following a traumatic event, I spent two years attempting to heal through therapy, but to no avail. My daily life was plagued by constant flashbacks, melancholy, and sorrow.

Fortunately, Ms. Brinkpeter guided me to escape the pervasive negative thought cycle that had ensnared me for far too long.

Remarkably, after just one session, I noticed an immediate improvement—a truly wonderful feeling. This sense of well-being only grew in the subsequent days, making me eager for our next session utilizing the Simpson Protocol.

Through learning self-hypnosis, I've become impervious to what used to trigger me. Currently, I'm enjoying a newfound sense of joy and a dramatically transformed mindset. Ms. Brinkpeter's assistance has been transformative, and I am profoundly grateful for my rejuvenated state of well-being. My heartfelt thanks to you, Birgit. **Andrea Zimmer**

I highly endorse this to anyone facing similar challenges. I was once debilitated by panic attacks to the extent that enduring car rides for over an hour seemed insurmountable. As I pen this review from my summer retreat in Noordwijk, it's a testament to the transformative power of the Simpson Protocol and Ms. Brinkpeter's guidance. This experience has rekindled my zest for life. My gratitude towards you is boundless! **Lisa Brunke**

I've had a chance to experience Birgit's gifts and light that she is bringing for others. Absolutely beautiful, thank you for your service. **Nikoleta Zolner**

Birgit Alaya Brinkpeter   birgit@happy-hypnoses.de

NOTE Ines Simpson

This process of therapy that became Simpson Protocol was a journey in experimentation to make things easier and simpler for the Client and the Practitioner

Jerry Kein said all Practitioners need to experiment 10% of the time – otherwise we just keep repeating old tropes. And as Hypnosis is not open-heart surgery - you can't hurt anyone – the worst that can happen is you think – well that's didn't do anything let's do this.

I wanted to find a process that didn't need the Client to have to relive Trauma experiences to get rid of them. And a process that I could use when the Client really didn't want to tell me the issue – just wanted me to somehow 'fix' it. With the caveat – the Client still had to be open to doing 'the work' in the process.

So, SP became a process, where you the Practitioner didn't need to know the issue the Client brought you, and you didn't need a different 'script' for every issue.

SP empowers the Client to work through their issues in a simple safe and easy fashion – and come through the process clear and free.

The key words in SP – Can we do now everything that is Appropriate, Beneficial and Optimum for this client at this time.

Chapter 2- Coming Home

BELGIUM and HOLLAND

NOTE Ines Simpson

Originally the key areas for SP in Europe were Belgium, Netherlands, Germany and France. And it has moved out from there.

In each case this was because of the amazing SP Trainers who work in those areas.

Germany of course is Stin-Niels Musche as mentioned, and France has Ludovic Louissaint, who you will meet in the next section.

Belgium/Netherlands SP is all because of Christophe Dierckx

When Stin-Neils Musche took over the training in Germany, I was looking for other places where SP would be welcomed.

As I was born in Belgium, I really wanted to work SP into Belgium. I always felt an affinity for Belgium when I visited there.

It started in The Netherlands.

I knew an Omni a trainer based in the Netherlands and at a Swiss Convention we talked about setting up an SP Training in Holland, which she promptly did.

Stin and I drove up there from Germany and had our first training with about 20 students.

One of those students was Christophe Dierckx from Zandhoven near Antwerp. And he was staying in the same hotel as I was, and we connected. Plus, he offered to give me rides back and forth to the hotel. A bonus!

At some point before I left, we discussed with Christophe the possibility of him becoming the SP trainer for Belgium and Holland. At that point it was just an idea.

When I was back in Canada, I approached Rob de Groof in Aarschott, Belgium as he has a Hypnosis training school there, and is always looking for extra courses for his students. And so, we set an SP training in Aarschot, Belgium.

Hey SP in Belgium!

(Plus, it gave me an excuse to visit Bruges again.)

Christophe came to that training, and then he came to the first SP German Birthing training we had in Hamburg. And we were set.

Christophe had many doubts about making SP training work for him in Belgium and Holland – starting from zero. But he has made Dutch a key language for SP, and the Belgium/ Dutch SP'ers have added so much to the SP process.

Christophe, himself, has become an amazing Hypnotist and teacher. And he has done things that would perhaps be considered miracles outside of SP.

His belief and trust in SP is second to none. And as with all the great trainers and Practitioners we have – he has moved SP forward again and again.

As he said to me one time – *"its amazing – imagine if you could connect with a 'Wisdom' (the SuperConscious Mind) and not only receive wisdom – but you can talk to the wisdom and receive the answers you need- incredible."*

Christophe Dierckx, SP Trainer – Belgium and Holland

I sat in the shade at the back of the garden on a chair under the Linden tree. It was a Friday afternoon, and Tanja was in the hammock and already in a trance. Several months earlier, Ines Simpson had asked me to experiment with "ultra." The guides of guides. She knew I liked to explore new things with hypnosis. She said, "Christophe, you check from your side that it is safe to work with "ultra" (not only with the SuperConscious Mind) and then we can start to teach in this as well.".

Since that day, I had already started working to connect with "ultra" in my hypnosis sessions at the end. Everything was ok. Clients thought it was a wonderfully positive experience. Some said it was strong or experienced a lot of light. Therefore, I had asked Tanja to devote an entire session to "ultra". She can speak well in trance, which sometimes makes things easier than just working with yes/no feedback.

From the time Tanja was in the state of "high," I asked if a connection could be made to "ultra".

The answer was, "Of course!"

When asked if it was safe and ok, I got positive answers every time.

When I asked "ultra": "Who are you anyway?", I got the following answer... "Christophe, you know best who I am".

I answered laconically: "I don't think so. Otherwise, I wouldn't have asked that question".

Immediately afterwards, Tanja changed her voice to a stern yet respectful tone:

Ultra said in her voice, "Your son will make a drawing. In that drawing, you will see the moon, the stars, and a planet. Through that drawing, you will know who I am!". And then the voice fell away.

 Tanja quietly returned from her trance and looked at me with big eyes as she said, "Wow, what energy."

Now, it was 2:30 pm. Tanja went home, and I took my bicycle to pick up the children (still small at the time) at school. I had just reached the playground, and Ruben (my little son) walked up to me with ... a drawing in his hands. It was a watercolour painting on cardboard. He had painted the moon, stars, and Uranus. And the teacher had stapled some notes to it. On those notes was the Genesis story. On Day 1, God separated light and darkness; on Day 2, God created the sky and water...

Tears rolled down my cheeks as I read this. Half an hour earlier, Tanja told me my son would draw a picture. Had I spoken to God? Since that day, my life has changed completely. Confidence in my holistic hypnosis work has gone through the roof. Thank you, Ines, for the confidence.

Christophe Dierckx <u>christophe.dierckx@icloud.com</u>

NOTE *Ines Simpson*: As you will see in the section with Justine Lette in New Zealand – Ultra became a major 'guide' for us in SP. And through that process we were introduced to many other 'guides/energies' that allowed SP to work in areas and with issues we have never touched before.

As with most things SP -it was a very connected event. Christophe mentioned he had been working in a session and this 'force, energy 'appeared a force for good – and said he could call him' Ultra' if he liked– names meant nothing to that energy.

A little while later Stin was talking to me and mentioned an energy that had taken over a session and created an amazing outcome for the client.

And then in a New Zealand class – Ultra paid me a visit, as you will read in Justine Lette's contribution.

INES SIMPSON – SP Group sessions

Nancy Schilder has great success with Group SP Sessions. In the SP Courses we teach how to conduct a Self-Hypnosis workshop – where you have a group experience SP Self Hypnosis, not only experience it – but also learn it for themselves so they can have Self Hypnosis self-care anywhere.

Heidi Puffing in Austria also specialized in SP group sessions and has found great success with them.

SP Group sessions can be with two or three participants in groups of 80 people and more.

Justine Lette (SP Trainer N.Z Australia) and Christophe and I did an online group workshop for more than 80 people. And I met one of the participants a while later and asked her – how was it with such a large group. She said – "well for me – I thought it was just me there! "

Nancy Schilder, SP Practitioner

Netherlands

Every time I do a Simpson session I am surprised by the impact on people. That is why I decided to do group sessions so I could make it more affordable for people AND help more people at a time.

Because of the group size I can't always follow everyone with their 'Yes' and their 'No' so I just ask Higher Consciousness and guidance to do the full job. And every time it works.

People feel the biggest shifts and I can feel those shifts in the room too.

People come into these sessions with all manner of issues.

From a person with a frozen shoulder (they couldn't lift up their arm before the session, and after the session it moved with ease) to a person with really high anxiety levels that was so happy the way she felt after the session, she decided to tell everyone in her neighborhood!

 My daughter was never able to go to the toilet outside of her home for a poop. When I did a huge group session during my volunteer work as a chiropractor in Haiti, and most of the group (80+ people divided into 2 sessions) joined in, she sat in too.

Recently she told me laughing that after this session she can do it anywhere now (imagine my relief!).

When a colleague in that same volunteer group asked for another session, I did another small group session with her and 2 other people.

Again, the shifts in that room were palpable.

They all went into an unwinding (your body starts to move to release the tension), not knowing that they were all doing the same thing. At the end of that volunteer work the lady who asked for a 2nd session told me that the 2 sessions she did with me did more than years of psychological and psychotherapy work. The others also mentioned it was a huge change they felt in their body.

I also did a 1-on-1 session with a client of another chiropractor in Venice, Italy. The lady client wanted to quit smoking and so my colleague told her to contact me. I never learned smoking protocol in hypnotherapy, so I just decided that part of the sessions was going to be Simpson. One session via Zoom and the lady was done with smoking.

My colleague did a shout out to me on Facebook for everyone to see to say thank you and how amazing this was. Not that I need a pat on the back, but this was really nice of her. The client got back to me after about a month and told me there has not been an urge to take out a cigarette anymore.

Although I know it works, it keeps on surprising me every time how special this protocol is. I just love it.

Nancy Schilder nancy@natuurlijkchiropractie.nl

SP CHINA via Belgium

Zhi Yang- SP Trainer Mandarin

My name is Zhi Yang (杨智), I am a devoted mother to Louis and Theo and married to my Belgian husband Alof.

My professional journey has thrived in Antwerp, Belgium, over two decades, where I explored marketing and sales across diverse industries after completing my master's studies.

Yet, beyond the confines of the corporate world, my lifelong quest was for life's purpose, truth, and self-understanding began in childhood.

Fascinated by biography books from middle school through university, each life story imparted profound lessons.

Curiously, my fascination extended to hypnosis books in my late twenties, igniting an unexpected passion. Through these readings, I recognized the immense potential of hypnosis—an instrument not just to unlock individual lives but the vast reservoirs of human consciousness.

As if completing a puzzle, years of inner calling culminated in a serendipitous encounter—the day I met SP founder Ines Simpson. And from there I embraced SP.

My online training in September 2021 marked a transformative shift—from a curious seeker to a dedicated SP practitioner committed to guiding my clients.

Attaining the title of SP Trainer for Chinese (Mandarin) became a milestone, garnering trust within the SP community and further responsibilities.

My joy stems from witnessing the transformative power of SP, not only within myself but also within my family and clients.

As Ines always explains, it's always a choice.

And it's my choice to embrace a path rich in learning, experiences, and positivity—a journey extended to my clients and SP colleagues alike.

I have found SP to be a great process to work not just with the individual – but also with couples.

With every session, the profound impact unveils the inherent potential within each individual.

I am excited to offer SP as a transformative tool, empowering others towards a more fulfilling life—a choice I make daily.

Zhi Yang – if you want change – consider changing yourself first.

I grew up in a relatively positive environment with guidance and attention, while my Husband came from a completely opposite environment, which brought loads of trauma and negative habits.

These differences and challenges made our relationship and marriage very difficult for years in the beginning.

I often suggested to him that he should see a hypnotherapist, but, of course, he ignored it. As you know, in a marriage, the best way to improve is to change yourself, not your partner.

So, one day, I decided to thoroughly discover and change myself. I received three sessions from Ines and learned SP myself.

My husband was curious, but I was careful not to rush things. Patience is key.

I offered a session, didn't insist, and just let him take his own time, but he was willing to try. And even after a few sessions – the dark side of him came out less and less.

Here, I need to emphasize that even if you're the best therapist in the world, you cannot push your partner if they are not ready!

The amazing thing about SP is that the client doesn't need to tell you anything, and it works!

Now my husband feels more and more at ease and remains calm no matter what the situation would have previously triggered him. Thanks to SP, he has also been able to develop hobbies that bring him happiness.

I take a moment sometimes to look back at where our joint journey originated and observe where it is now and imagine where it will be.

I constantly feel that my husband is so wise, and actually, it's always he who guides me instead.

Who guides whom, who knows.

The journey of each individual is completely different, and in our case, or as in any other, real joy always comes from within, not from your partner.

I am happy that he gave himself the opportunity to experience SP. Starting from there, he has become a more loving father to our two boys, a more understanding husband, and most importantly, he is more positive and pursuing his own inner journey in his unique way.

Couples Therapy-Zhi Yang

Sometimes, you suddenly comprehend why life has bestowed upon you certain experiences and led you to where you are; similarly, when the universe brought me, numerous clients grappling with relationship difficulties.

Drawing from my personal experience and utilizing the tool of SP, one of my services is, I assist individual clients and couples seeking deeper connections within their current relationships or marriages.

Using hypnosis as a technique, they empower themselves to tap into their inner strength and discover themselves or enhance their long-term relationships.

My joy stems from witnessing their success moments, whether they arrive at these realizations consciously or during our sessions and observe them progressively embracing positivity within their relationships or marriages.

Key elements in this transformative journey are forgiveness and understanding, and of course with SP, it's much easier.

Zhi Testimonials

Olga, Netherlands

I found myself in the middle of a nasty divorce and had completely lost myself. I was struggling with my new reality as a single mom of two and the pain and emotions that came with it all.

I met Zhi, and she spoke to me about the hypnotherapy she did and how she could help me heal from past trauma, give me strength, and reset my goals in life by speaking to my super conscious mind.

I found this interesting and needed some help to give me a new direction in life, so I decided to follow a couple of sessions with her.

It gave me guidance in my new life, brought me back into balance, and helped me reach my new goals and enjoy life again.

Now, a year later, I am so much happier and can deal with my emotions so much better. I achieved my first goals, which were two certifications in child psychology and child coaching, which gave me back my confidence.

You must do the work yourself, but the hypnotherapy sessions by Zhi helped me to push myself in the right direction, and I can enjoy life and see a great future for myself and my kids again.

Ilke, Belgium

I came to Zhi after a suggestion from the osteopath I went to for pain in my neck and shoulders.

The concrete trigger was my the very deep-seated fear of surgery by the dentist. I had to have a front tooth extracted and replaced with an implant because there had been inflammation on the root for over 20 years.

The problem with my tooth dates to when I was about 6 years old and learning to ride a bike. My dad was holding my bike and walking behind me, and the moment he let go and yelled, "You can do it! You are off on your own!"

I fell flat on my face causing my front tooth to fall out....

I had long felt that there was a connection between that fall 35 years ago and my current fear of getting that tooth treated at the dentist. It was literally and figuratively about getting to the root of the problem.

In addition to the fear of the dentist that was evident on the surface, I was also dealing with a deeper fear that I did not initially express to Zhi. Not because of a lack of trust in her but for fear of making the fear even bigger and more real by expressing it.

I sat with the fear of having to leave my partner. A kind of - very irrational - reverse separation anxiety that went very deep and at times had a gigantic impact on my daily functioning – such as not being able to sleep, no appetite, uncontrollable crying fits....

In the three hypnosis sessions I had with Zhi, the fear on these two levels was addressed and transformed.

I still went to the dentist with clammy hands but after all these years of putting it off, it was a gigantic victory to take this step. With the help of the self-hypnosis exercise plus a sedative pill and the presence of my partner, I was in the dental chair with confidence.

The entire procedure went smoothly and prosperously, and as always with such things, I asked myself afterwards what I had been so afraid of all this time anyway!

What has changed after this procedure - besides the appearance of my smile - is the following: I got rid of the oppressive feeling that used to overwhelm me, a feeling I have had since I was a six-year-old girl.

Regarding the anxiety in my relationship, I benefited very much from what came out of the second hypnosis session. It showed that this life is currently the sixth reincarnation in which my partner and I are connected. I find it such a comforting idea that our souls chose - out of love - for each other to work something out together in this life.

Our two children were also there in five previous lives. The message from my unconscious that there is nothing to be afraid of helped me like a mantra when I felt fear bubbling back up afterwards.

I am very grateful for what the hypnosis sessions have brought me.

And so much depends on the way Zhi works.

She exudes great calm and wisdom. And you know she is with you, on your side.

The confidence she exudes to her clients is contagious!

Meanwhile, the last hypnosis session has been behind me for a while, and I am gradually daring to trust that the fear in my relationship is gone.

Occasionally I still feel the fear rearing its head. I think "that's ok – come on in"

 I then let her in, thank her kindly for her attentiveness and care for me but also tell her that I don't need her now because everything is under control...and so she can leave again!

Xiaomin, China

I have always been inexplicably interested in the meaning of life, religion, and supernatural powers/energies.

With each experience in my life where things went as I wished, I also experienced moments of emptiness, powerlessness, and confusion. I am aware that there is a very high-dimensional consciousness behind humanity, but I feel very chaotic and lost.

Zhi is one of the few friends with whom I can deeply discuss such soul topics.

When she obtained her qualification as a SP hypnotherapist, I was very lucky and excited to be one of her first few experiencers in the Chinese session.

During the experience, she guided me, and my Mind led me into a world of dazzling white light, where I merged into the light, feeling as if there was nothing else present, and the boundaries of time and space seemed to disappear. At the end of the session, I did no feeling of change – at that time. However, changes gradually manifested over time.

I found myself having more opportunities and moments of awareness from a conscious perspective, spending more time in a positive state of mind, and gradually gaining clarity in direction.

I also found myself connecting more frequently with people and content of higher energy, feeling more relaxed and at ease, and gradually discovering the direction and purpose of my life.

I am grateful to Zhi for awakening my ability to connect with the supernatural energy of my higher self. I am even more grateful for Zhi's spiritual companionship, bringing nourishment to my soul and abundance to my spiritual life.

I believe that with Zhi's guidance, you, and countless others can achieve peace, harmony, joy, and freedom in life. Zhi can lead us on a journey that is both interesting and meaningful. Are you ready?

Zhi Yang info@zhihypnosis.com　　　　www.zhihypnosis.com

Liesbeth Meuldijk – de Jong, SP Practitioner

The Netherlands

I am Liesbeth Meuldijk, a Certified Simpson Protocol Practitioner in Holland. I like to tell you about SP, because for me Simpson Protocol is one of the most beautiful opportunities for inner growth. It brought me a gift for life, so I learned all levels and became a Certified SP Practitioner. Here is my story, I hope it may inspire you.

Since I started working as a hypnotherapist (2017), the power of hypnosis keeps surprising me. It is a soft and effective way to ask the unconscious mind for help, because it contains all the right information to solve problems. That is why my guidance is always aimed at identifying and removing causes, so the annoying symptoms will also disappear.

When I was told about SP, I directly recognized the possibilities Wow... what an incredibly special and loving hypnosis method! What a wonderful idea to receive help from an own higher mindpower, which has special, sincere, and pure intentions and can connect you to everything. All humans have this inner, intuitive, and self-healing source since they started their life. It is protective, will know the right answers, gives information, and does never say "yes" to something that will be harmful to that person. With SP, you can learn how to trust your self-healing abilities better, by understanding that your smart and clever brain part can do far more work than you ever thought would be possible. Because it is precisely by understanding our thoughts, traumas, and blockages, it can offer you a chance for optimal recovery on all levels.

The life of every human being begins as soon as the soul descends into an embryo in the mother's womb. Without a soul, life is impossible.   It is my believe that souls can have history, can be carrying traumas and attachments or that they can lose a soul part. I find it interesting to find out how people are put together, how their souls work, how they are consciously and unconsciously shaped in their thinking, acting, and feeling

by positive and negative emotions and events. How each small or large unpleasant experience from the very beginning can deeply anchored and later felt, causing all kinds of complaints, without any memory. These emotions and feelings can be like a tree with several roots, connecting to any kind of cause.

Babies can hear and feel in the womb, so all events during mother's pregnancy up to early childhood can have effect. At higher age, you can feel something is strange or missing inside, without being able to articulate or tell what that is exactly. But we humans also know there is only one brain inside. A person's brain sends information to its own body by means of all kinds of thoughts and impulses. Also, Highly Sensitive People are more aware of negative entities and external impulses in their feelings. If you are now thinking "how is this possible, I did not choose to have my troubles" you are right. Of course, complaints are no conscious choice or wish. Good news to know that SP can help you to solve a lot of your issues.

In conclusion: a brain controls the shell in which the brain is connected to (its own body) and at the same time this brain can perceive that such impulses cause complaints. The good news is that your subconscious remembers EVERYTHING that has happened in your life. Therefore, it is the best resource to apply for information. It is especially important to discover your unconscious level and be more aware how you influenced yourself and your body, by accepting help from all available universal and higher sources out of trust.

The SELF-HYPNOSIS method of Simpson Protocol is based on SELF-LOVE. How we humans influence our mind and body, the mirror of the brain, OURSELVES. There were already various methods of help, hypnosis types, books, NLP, and more. All that fascinating information remains interesting to absorb and apply. Yet, any change will only take place when you really allow yourself to do so, deep within, thus giving you a chance to change and renew. And if it is needed, you just ask for support and guidance to take the right step and open up to what will present itself.

This is the secret that sets the Simpson Protocol apart from other methods. It uses the greatest and purest resource that exists, which is already present IN people. Simpson Protocol comes from universal LOVE, which is all-encompassing and healing. A pure source that will always be there for you if you so desire. And no matter how many success stories you will read: only when you experience this unique protocol yourself will you understand what we, all writers, mean....

My first SP gave me that special feeling. My clients know it, felt it. Self-help through Self-love through Self-hypnosis with Simpson Protocol. Do you want to experience this? I will be happy to help you and hope to see you.

Happy regards from   **Liesbeth Meuldijk – de Jong**

www.blijvanbinnen.nl   www.happyinsidehypnosis.nl

Hanne Essers, SP Practitioner

Mol, Belgium

As a child, I regularly heard that I was so sweet, quiet, and patient. Nice to hear, so I made every effort to keep those "titles". But it began to gnaw... more and more. I noticed restlessness inside, frustration, sometimes even outright anger. And I didn't even know why! I couldn't do anything with it either. Breaking something was a waste and would only cause more pain in my body.

Screaming out loud didn't suit my feelings. It never relieved either. And believe me, I tested it many times. I just couldn't do it...

It almost seemed like I was carrying around an anger that didn't belong to me, a kind of ghost hanging around me when I knew so well that ghosts don't exist.

Until I discovered in a session SP that there were indeed entities with me. And not the Casper-the-friendly-spooky kind... They were angry, raging even!

And there, suddenly, out of nowhere and still full of disbelief... I learned to guide these 'ghosts' to where they did belong, in all love and with the utmost respect. For sweet, calm, and patient I was apparently still... Whew!

Gone was the anger, gone was the frustration, gone was also the search for how to express my anger. I didn't have to express anything; it just wasn't even mine!

Coming home after the session, my husband asked, "Gee, what happened to you? Your eyes are shining brighter than ever!"

Bright! ... that was the nail on the head. 'Ghosts' do exist, and oh how sweet they are, once you know how to deal with them!

SP changed my life. From anger to peace, from fear to confidence, from disbelief to acceptance and from intense grief during a grieving process to a beautiful connection full of gratitude.

In short, I wish everyone to experience the endless possibilities of SP... Even if you are still thinking it doesn't exist!

Hanne Essers - Flow of mind- info@flowofmind.be

Miranda Geens, SP Practitioner

Betekom, Belgium

Some case Studies

A lady came to me to lose weight because the dietician is not helping. After a third session, the lady asks what I did to her the previous session because she was supposed to have surgery on her wrist but after a checkup just before the surgery, the specialist told her with surprise that it was no longer necessary, her wrist was healed.

I do remember that in that particular session, the lady (I was completely unaware of the wrist problem) during the session indicated that her wrist hurt, she was also very cold.

Meanwhile, the lady is also quietly losing weight. And she changed jobs, and her husband tells me - she looks happy again.

A young woman of 27 came to me as she could barely keep her job, barely stay at work.

She told me she had lactose intolerance, fibromyalgia, fatigue, burnout, panic attacks, heart palpitations, and so on.

In addition, she has a boyfriend who actually uses her when it suits him.

So, we begin some SP sessions.

After a few sessions she sent me a message that her boyfriend broke up with her. She wasn't the same anymore he told her, of course she was now standing up for herself more and more which he didn't like.

We continued to work, and the girl kept taking steps forward, she changed jobs, became more assertive, stopped being dependent on the infirmary, had less pain, had more energy, changed jobs again and could gradually eat chocolate, cheese, sauce yes even cake again.

The panic attacks were as good as gone and when one did start sputtering, she managed to control them very quickly. Meanwhile, she has a new boyfriend and is very happy. The sessions continued every 3 to 4 weeks because it was felt that the changes in her body needed time to adjust, so yes this took six months, but what a change.

An anorexia patient of 14 years old, she was written off everywhere, dietician, therapy, psychologists, osteopaths, yes even hospitalizations, nothing helped, the parents were desperate and came to me by word of mouth.

Knowing what SP can do – I thought this would be a simple process.

But as in any Hypnosis session, you can't force someone into hypnosis, and this girl did not want to be helped.

And after a few chats – I sensed the mother too was losing hope.

So first gaining trust with the girl was necessary and gaining an understanding of her situation.

The girl was the oldest of 3 sisters, always very well behaved, obedient... while the other sister had tantrums and therefore enjoyed the necessary attention and the youngest sister 'because she was the youngest', also received a lot of attention.

To put it briefly, the girl was now also getting attention because of her eating disorder. The causes came out very clearly, she knew how to tell the situation very clearly. Now that we knew the causes we could continue to work. I was finally able to help her with a mix of talks, listening ear and SP.

A lady of 72 who ended up in a burn-out asked for my help. Psychiatrist, two months of institutionalization, several psychologists, group discussions...nothing could help her.

She too came to me; I can still see her coming in as a wreck and very emaciated. In the sessions many issues came up about 'burn out', such as not yet having gotten over the death of her parents, parents-in-law, brother, son-in-law, such as bullying during her youth, never being allowed to continue her studies.

Through this session this lady is now much calmer, starting to make herself beautiful again, to make up, she is regaining her appetite, etc... We are not quite there yet, but the once negative lady enters the practice smiling.

Miranda Geens   miranda.geens@telenet.be

Corrie van Pinxteren, SP Practitioner

Netherlands

Using Surrogate Hypnosis

SP Surrogate Hypnosis is when the Practitioner works through a Surrogate to the Client. The client will usually be unaware of the ongoing process (but not the outcome). And it only works if the SuperConscious say yes you may connect their Higher Minds – at the highest level.

In this case Corrie was both the Surrogate and Practitioner

My story is about Jasper and his father Ron.

In May 2021, Jasper and his mother came to me for the first session. Jasper suffers suffering from complex compulsions, actions and thoughts. Jasper is mildly mentally limited and has autism.

For this he has been under treatment at various youth health organizations and hospitals from 2013 to 2017.

Jasper is obsessed with his appearance with a focus on how his hair sits and feels. He is of the opinion that his hair is terrible and that he really cannot go outside with this or go to school with it. He is not allowed to sit down by himself -only when he eats or drink- so he just keeps walking around in circles.

He cannot/will not go into the garden alone and always wants someone to go with him. He finds watching TV difficult, this is tied to all kinds of rules and also with his phone there are compulsions. He is angry, frustrated and does not want to not want to go on living like this.

Before the session I discussed with his mother that I do not know how many sessions I will need, but that I will do everything in consultation with what we call the SuperConscious.

After the preliminary conversation with Jasper during the first session, I decided to treat Jasper with SP Surrogate Hypnosis through myself.

When the session is over, Jasper is just disappointed. He feels nothing, has only been lying quietly on the couch; in short, nothing has changed. He grumbles in the car home and repeatedly asks his mother if she wants to drive the car into a tree. To turn everything to the positive, his mother decides to give him a treat him to a snack at the gas station; this will become a tradition after every session.

In the days that follow, Jasper notices that things are changing, and when he visits me again a few weeks after that he visits me again, he is excited, as he notices the changes in himself.

He can sit down anywhere; he doesn't have to do all kinds of all kinds of compulsive actions on his phone or on the television.

After each session Jasper and those around him notice changes, he also notices that compulsions go away but also that new compulsions arise.

After consulting with his mother, we decided to start working with SP Surrogate Hypnosis through her from now on.

In the period that Jasper has sessions with me, in October 2022 Jasper's father becomes seriously ill, there are tumors in his head. He is forgetful, cannot think of words, sits lifeless in a chair, gets stuck in computer and chore actions he undertakes nothing anymore and is incontinent.

The prognosis is that he has 3 months to live.

Together all decided to start the sessions immediately and that we will also do them with SP Surrogate Hypnosis. Ron and Claudia want to go on a cruise with their children and so we decided to start the sessions as soon as possible.

I discussed with Christophe Dierckx, the Belgian SP Trainer, how to best use SP surrogacy in this case.

During the session I do not speak of a tumor but of a swelling. In the first session I ask if the swelling consists of several parts, and it does. I name it as 'swelling 1' and 'swelling 2', in all the sessions that follow I continue to do so.

The SuperConscious indicates that we should treat the swellings separately.

We do a total of 4 sessions of 2 hours in 6 days.

The first two were at my office, the other two online.

After the first two sessions there are already small changes. When we take a break after the third session and Claudia walks into the living room, Ron has already done some work, hung paintings and done something in the garden.

In short, he is very busy. He also filled out the forms on the computer, filled out the forms for the cruise they are going to take in the next week.

Claudia is afraid that they will not be able to enjoy it fully, and especially she dreads the plane ride they will have to take before the cruise.

The attending specialist has also advised Ron against flying at this time.

 They would like to have these beautiful memories with both sons and decide to go anyway.

I agree with her that during the cruise I will keep everything as optimal for Ron as possible for me.

We start the fourth session; in the last few days we have worked through all the issues regarding the swellings.

Now we look to see if any other organs are involved or compromised.

During this session, I myself go into a kind of trance. It didn't last long, but I began to say things out loud and addressed my client by another name: Frank.

When I came out of the trance, I did not really know what had happened. I was very tired and needed some time to recover myself.

I asked Ron, to confirm, "did I call you by another name in that session?" "Yes" he says "you called me Frank".

So then with Ron in Hypnosis, I ask "Superconscious does Frank have anything to do with this session?" to which I received a "Yes."

 "SuperConscious, may I ask why Frank is coming to this session?"

To which my client under hypnosis replies, "Frank is coming to help the process -Frank will make sure that s everything will be optimal in this process."

And by the way, as far as I know, to this day, Frank is still there to help him.

Now because Ron and Claudia are anxious about the upcoming trip

– we have a session to work on the fears and issues surrounding this trip.

In the session SuperConscious links the colour Green as an anchor to be used during the trip.

(an anchor is a word, or symbol, or in this case Colour, that is used to bring back calm, balance and harmony if any anxiety, in this case, arises)

The family travels towards the airport, everyone is wearing something green except Jasper.

He didn't like that and quickly bought a nice green shirt at the airport.

The flight went smoothly, and they all greatly enjoyed the cruise, Ron especially.

In our subsequent sessions – the SuperConscious indicated there would be support for Ron and Jasper at all times,

Jasper went into assisted living in December 2022. It can be quite challenging for him. But he uses his triggers when a compulsion is developing and can mostly keep things under control.

If there is a need, we work together with an SP Hypnosis session.

Just before the summer vacation in 2023 it seemed that one of Ron's swellings had grown, a discoloration could be seen on the photos.

We had a session, and in the session, SuperConscious indicated that there was no growth, and all would be well.

We are one year and four months on. Ron is doing well, dealing with Jasper is improving after each session. He is involved, does chores in and around the house and does not suffer from incontinence.

It is an honor for me to do this together with Claudia for Ron and Jasper.

Corrie van Pinxteren Resilience Counseling & Therapy Nistelrode NL

Marianne Eelen SP Practitioner

Belgium

Case 1

Together with a fellow student, we planned to practice some SP online. It was one of our first practice sessions ever. I didn't know anything to work on and with the thought in mind that you should be open to possibilities, I suggested working on my frozen shoulder. And so, my practice partner did.

My shoulder had already been blocked for more than a year. Although I was already going twice a week to the physiotherapist, I didn't make any progress... I still couldn't undo or fasten my bra at my back: in fact, I couldn't even touch the clasp of it because I couldn't get my left arm higher than my waistband.
After the session, I felt as if I had fallen asleep during the session. I

was completely unaware of what happened, except for the end. I heard that it would take six weeks to process the session. To follow up on the result, I had written that date in my agenda.

During the fifth week I could already touch the clasp of my bra at the back of my back with my left hand. This was already very remarkable since I was already used to opening and closing my bra in front of me. And exactly six weeks later, I could open it at the back of back without any effort or pain.

I was completely amazed and even found it terrifying: does God really exist then?

In one of the next practice sessions, my fellow student took me to "Divine". Just one sentence: "Please, bring her to Divine" … and I felt instantly this very deep bliss; tears were rolling on my face…

That my frozen shoulder was cured by hypnosis is one thing, but that the prediction of the process was perfectly correct, left me completely in awe.

We are now 2 1/2-year son. The pain and blockage in my shoulder never came back.

Case 2

About a year and a half ago, I suddenly had hot flashes, waking up totally sweaty… Seemed to be menopausal…

Brought myself to Peace, Deep and High and asked if SCM could solve this issue with the subliminal technique. It was a "Yes". So I did.

I didn't have any hot flashes for more than a year. They immediately stopped.

A few months ago, they were back.

I did again the subliminal technique in self-hypnosis asking for a comfortable body temperature. Processing time would be 2 weeks. And that was true. I have no hot flashes or sweaty nights anymore.

(subliminal is a way in SP Hypnosis for the Conscious Mind to know the session has been completed)

Case 3

My dearest aunt was 85 years old and had lost the use of her kidneys.

For 15 years she had been going to Kidney Dialysis 3 times a week.

Then during the Pandemic, she contracted the COVID 19 Virus and was put into Hospital.

When she finally left hospital, she was very weak.

Her blood values were very bad, she really looked very bad (as someone on her deathbed) and the doctors decided that, from now, she had to have 4 kidney dialysis per week.

She not only looked like someone on her deathbed, but she also felt like someone on her deathbed. She said: "you don't have to wash my socks anymore because I will be dead the end of this week..."

That night I did a very short self-hypnosis surrogacy session with only the subliminal technique.

My hand was moving like crazy, on its own, uncontrollable, until my arm dropped. 5 days later, I visited my aunt again.

I brought my harp, since I knew this was one of her last wishes to play the harp.

Yet she looked completely different, the death mask was gone, she looked fully happy again and the doctor tested her blood again the day after I did the self-surrogacy SP: her blood values were okay. She had to go "only" 3 times per week to the kidney dialysis.

1 year later she decided to stop the dialysis, and she died 1 week later.

The week after, I followed the Spirit SP class with Lance Baker, and I was chosen to be in the demo.

I connected with my aunt, and I really felt her presence and the bliss she was living in the afterlife.

This helped me so much to cope with the loss of my beloved aunt. For me, she is still alive and very close to me.

The concept of death has completely changed for me.

Marianne Eelen eelenmarianne@gmail.com

INES SIMPSON *Language and Code words*

In this work we are using the parts of us that have no language.
And yet to access those parts we use language.

So, in SP the language must be open and as a student said artfully
vague. Vague so we don't box anything in (and lock things out) and
artful to still get the right approach without the exact words.

This is done with what we call code words and Intention.

Code words are words like SuperConscious, Depth of the State,
Spirit, Soul, Chakras, and so on. Even the word we use for the
Client's situation – we call it 'the issue'. So, it's not one thing, but
whatever is being worked on – and we never know what is being
worked on – because we are not doing the work, and the conscious
mind is not doing the work.

Words that can attract the meaning required by the person at that
time for that issue.

But also, with intention – the practitioner always holds the
intention of creating the most Optimum, Beneficial, and
Appropriate outcome for this client at this time.

Language is important – especially in places that have no language.

Chapter 3-- Bonjour au Protocole Simpson Français

NOTE Ines Simpson

As I have said the key areas for SP in Europe are Belgium/Netherlands, Germany and France. In each case this is because of the amazing SP Trainers who work in those areas.

Germany of course is Stin-Niels Musche as mentioned, Belgium/Netherlands is because of Christophe Dierckx who you met in the last section. And France has Ludovic Louissaint.

Ludovic had emailed me about a training I was doing in London UK – the first 4 day Training I had done there.

Previously we did 2 days of training and then came back within 6 months to do 2 more days of what at that time was called "Advanced SP Training."

He emailed me to ask if I thought it would be ok, as his English was not that great – though looking at his emails- I wasn't sure why he was concerned.

Anyway, I told him, when you are using SuperConscious to do the work – language was not an issue – and this work was done in a place where language was irrelevant.

Thankfully, he decided to turn up.

Ludovic impressed me immediately - he is a very smart hypnotist Practitioner/Psychologist and caught on very quickly in class.

And, small aside, he had the female section of that class smiling – a lot!

SP at that time was emphasizing Esdaile as the state to attain and work from – nowadays we find it is no longer needed, but from Esdaile we found it was easy to move to the deeper level of Sichort – and maintain connection to the client. And Esdaile is used in SP now for Pain control or relief, especially in things like the SP Birthing program.

As Ludovic says he came to learn this 'mysterious' technique SP has which was not just being able to have the client achieve Esdaile very easily and quickly, but also maintain communication, through Ideomotor response at the Esdaile level.

Of course, the first demo I did within the first half hour demonstrated Esdaile and communication with a volunteer student – and as he says – he thought it would take all the 4 days of training to learn this Esdaile technique – and it was done in the first 20 minutes, and then in every practice the students themselves did that morning!

Ludovic, as have so many SP practitioners, has helped to take SP to another level. His trust and belief in the concept of the Subconscious, and the process with the client has allowed him to do amazing things with SP.

If you Google Ludovic on YouTube and check out his YouTube channel - you will see some of the remarkable things he does with SP- on a daily basis.

Ludovic Louissaint - SP Trainer – French

I am a Clinical Psychologist with a background in Neuropsychology.

I also trained in brief therapy and EMDR. During my training, I had the opportunity to learn about Ericksonian hypnosis. A form of hypnosis I didn't like, as I found it too complicated and vague.

I then discovered Elmanian hypnosis with Jerry Kein, and that changed my vision of things. I went on to explore the Esdaile and the Ultra Height states.

I was having some difficulty with the Esdaile state, and while doing some research on the Internet, I stumbled across Ines Simpson and her Protocol. A little skeptical about achieving the Esdaile state for over 98% of clients in a single session, I signed up anyway.

And then ... everything changed in my practice, my belief system was turned upside down. My expectations were fulfilled after just 10 minutes (out of the 4 days of training). I did things I'd never even imagined possible.

As they say, serendipity plays its part.

I've lost count of the testimonials of phobias, anxiety attacks, PTSD, etc. released after 1 or 2 sessions so I'm not going to talk about them. I'm going to highlight some rather special sessions.

I'm seeing a young woman for the second time. The 1st was for work-related stress. We meet again 1 month later, and she tells me that she had to go to the emergency room because she had a panic attack at night as well as 4-5 similar attacks. Her companion found her with 2 hands on the cooking hobs (fortunately turned off), she woke up wanting to drink bleach, she woke up bleeding because she had scratched her arms, etc. Always in her sleep, without her being aware of it.

And she says to me "but I don't understand it, because since the last session, qualitatively, my life is better, even better".

(For reference, the 1st session was a classic).

At that moment, I had a flash. That of a deceased child...

So, I do what I never usually do, but I ask her (I usually avoid because I want to avoid suggestions): "Did your grandmother have a child death? But a premature or violent death?"

And then, to my great surprise, she says, "Yes, plenty. My grandmother had a lot of miscarriages, but I don't know more about it because it's a taboo subject. All I know is that my grandmother ended up developing bipolar disorder".

You start the session; something comes up that was emotional overload. Then comes the spiritual side. Bam a child comes. She tells me with fear "yes, it's him, it's a young boy, he's the one who's hurting me".

"SuperConscious, can she act as a channel?"

SuperConscious indicates "yes."

OK, go ahead and let this little boy express himself.

And then, it's terrible. His voice changes and he tells me he's sad and angry.

All in all, I'll give you the short version. The grandmother had an extramarital affair and wanted to get rid of the child (I didn't really understand whether he was born at 2 months or in utero at 2 months). He decided to haunt the grandmother and cause all the miscarriages. And to continue haunting the descendants so as not to be forgotten.

In fact, during the connection, my patient started crying, telling me: "I mustn't get pregnant, no child should have to go through this".

In the session, Superconscious 'freed' the little boy now my patient knows that she just must go to church to light 2 candles for him and not forget him. (I don't know why).

We'll see in 1 month what the results are, but then again, sometimes "weird" things can happen.

A lady suffering from diplopia (double vision) for several years following an optic nerve lesion. However, she came to work on her anxieties and the impact of other people's gaze.

 At the end of the session, I ask SuperConscious Mind, is there anything we can do for her eyesight? The SuperConscious answers "yes".

I simply ask it to do what it can, and once that's done, I ask the patient to open her eyes. And to my surprise, her condition had improved, and she was almost no longer seeing things twice.

I ask SuperConscious, "Can we release her completely? "

SuperConscious indicates "yes".

30 seconds later, my patient could see properly again.

A patient who came in to manage the pain of chronic shingles (which recurred every month). A single session of the Simpson Protocol was enough to free her not only from the pain, but also from the shingles...

A patient who had undergone knee replacement surgery. After 6 months of revalidation, she was still unable to move her leg. In the middle of a session, I asked the SCM, "Can you bend her leg?"

To my surprise, the leg bent by itself (indicating at the very least an emotional block). After 3 sessions, she was able to walk without crutches, drive and ride a bike. She retained some after-effects but was once again autonomous.

HERE ARE A FEW PATIENT TESTIMONIALS.

- It's been 3 days since my appointment with Mr. Louissaint ... After 10 years of anxiety, it's my first experience with hypnosis and I'm speechless ... to be seen in the long term but so far, I feel almost cured (part of me is afraid it's only temporary) but I'm hopeful I've never had even a day's respite before ... Mr. Louissaint is very professional, and I don't regret having chosen him.

- Hello, I feel that just one session has helped me enormously. My brain no longer thinks about the problem and when I want to think about it, I feel like it's telling me that it's no use and I feel like it's all gone. One session ... I was quite sceptical, and, in the end, you helped me enormously and I thank you for that. I had no idea hypnosis could be so magical. Thank you so much.

Feedback from an old patient.

What's great about your technique is that actually we have a choice. We have a choice to look at a memory with a different perspective. And that's what's great. You know I think that other therapeutic tools tend to limit the patient. They tend to control the patient to let him change his life but that's what limits him. He'll feel that his well-being will depend on those therapists his whole life. I think that it tends to make the patient a sort of addict to his therapist because he'll need someone else to resolve his issues.

Personally, when I came to you it was different. Since then, when I have an issue, I can do it myself (with self-hypnosis). I don't need anyone else. It's possible that something really really bad happens and then ... OK maybe I will not have the resources to do it myself and then I'll maybe need to do hypnosis with you one day.

That other kind of therapy can take 3-4 years or the whole life.

You know even if the change looks miraculous. Let's say If I go to Lourdes (in France), and I heal from a miracle, I will not think that this change comes from me. I will not think that I have the capability to manage my issues and my life.

And then my whole life, if something happens, I'll think that I need to go there again and pray. Without that I'm kinda screwed.

But with you it's different. You simply give us the keys for us to know how to do it to free ourselves from stuff. You gave me the keys to understanding myself, to listen to myself, to listen to the part of me that I didn't know existed. And so, I can do it myself, at home or my whole life and that's a great difference.

Ludovic Louissaint   ludovic.louissaint@gmail.com

Paul Arnaud, SP Practitioner

France

I'm a project manager with a Master's in IT, and I used to be CTO of one of the biggest Internet advertising agencies in France. Then I decided to take a different path in life. That's how I got into hypnosis, through a multidisciplinary approach, and then discovered deep hypnosis. In my practice, I've always been convinced that we have within us the keys to change; but more often than not, we don't know how to access them. When I first started using deep hypnosis, I either kept silent after asking the "inner healer" to do the work, or I used, more often than not, techniques tested by E.L. ROSSI.

As I continued my research into the different states of hypnosis, including the Esdaile state and the keys to accessing it revealed by D. Elman, I discovered Ines Simpson's approach. The protocol she created, based on what she found most effective, struck me as simple, appropriate, and non-intrusive. So, I naturally adopted it, knowing that it also puts the consultant before the practitioner.

What I like about SP is the absolute confidence in the consultant's ability to activate the responses that will enable him or her to move towards the well-being that suits him or her, while leaving the practitioner in the dark about what is being achieved. For me, it's essential not to say, "this is what you should do, or this is where you should go".

The only open question I ask at the beginning of the session is "How can I help you?"

After that, it's up to the consultant to come up with the answers that will enable him or her to move towards greater well-being.

Learning, during the first session, the states of consciousness accessible through self-hypnosis, when the person consciously wishes it, which go from a state of connection with all parts of the mind to a state of elevation, are also a specificity of PS.

Some Case Studies

Two fairly recent cases come to mind. One about a consultant who comes for fear of spiders and the other about a consultant who comes for Psoriasis.

For the Psoriasis, the person comes to see me as a last hope," she tells me when she makes the appointment.

 She can't sleep any more and has to follow a medical treatment that she considers to be heavy, with no guarantee of efficacy.

She has doubts about medical treatments and doesn't want to follow what her doctors recommend.

We work on the problem and the SuperConscious explains to the conscious mind that the treatment is indispensable because it is beyond her capabilities.

What's more, the SuperConscious makes a deal with the consultant that, in exchange for the treatment, he'll make the pain acceptable. At the end of the session, the consultant confessed to me that she still felt her Psoriasis "present", but that she no longer had the pain she used to, and that she was willing to follow the medical treatment.

The second consultant, on Arachnophobia, is more striking in my eyes. After checking that there were no other fears, I worked according to the SP on the problem. The point here is not to focus on the fear itself, which is only the tip of the iceberg. So, I worked on "the issue" without knowing what it was.

During the session, the SuperConscious reveals that this fear is protecting something more important.

In fact, the SC informs me that this phobia protects a trauma linked to incest suffered between the ages of 4 and 8.

Knowing that SP is based on a relationship of trust and openness with the consultant, I ask the SuperConscious if all parties agree to continue with me.

The answer is no, even after a request for mediation. The SuperConscious expresses his willingness to work with a woman and informs the conscious mind. The SuperConscious then agrees to lower the intensity of the phobia from 8/10 to 5/10.

When the woman emerges, she explains that she's still afraid of spiders, but less so. I inform her that I'm not the right person to accompany her, as her SuperConscious doesn't want to work further with me; she confirms this too. She agrees to let me give her the contact details of a specialist psychologist.

During the two sessions, the consultants learned to go into different altered states on their own and with full awareness.

Paul-Arnaud email: paularnaudpy@gmail.com - **website:** paularnaudpy.com

Nicole Ah-Von, SP Practitioner.

France

The Simpson Protocol changed my life.

Ericksonian hypnosis did not reassure me to start practicing.

The Simpson Protocol leaves no room for doubt and fear of doing wrong: the supraconscious is my ally and that of the client, I am confident from the moment I set up.

The Simpson Protocol opened the doors to the spiritual for me. The universe, energies, chakras, dowsing, magnetism, clairvoyance... Since the Simpson protocol, my vibration rate has increased, my "gifts" too.

One evening in my bed, I began a session of the Simpson protocol in self-hypnosis to "do good for my body", but I fell asleep before the end... The super superconscious continued: the next day and since that night, my body rejects rich, fatty, sugary, industrial foods, alcohol, I simply cannot swallow them, like after gastroenteritis. Also, 2 kilos are gone.

The Simpson protocol made me lighter.

The Simpson Protocol has obviously changed the lives of my clients, with efficiency and humility. A client wishing to drive again after a serious car accident, in 3-4 sessions on this subject, has:

- Started driving again after 2 years of stopping

- Resumed sexual relations with her husband

- Stopped yelling at your children

- Forgiven her husband for a buried and found story of a hidden child

- Returned to a normal life

Thank you very much Inès! Gratitude! I mentally thank you every session. Thank you for this work, this community, thank you for creating the Simpson Protocol Without forgetting Raphaël Delvaux who introduced me to the Simpson protocol and Ludovic Louissaint who trained me.

nicole.ahvon@orange.fr

Laurence Chemin, SP Practitioner.

France

Attracted to psychology since adolescence, I wanted to go down this professional path, but came up against a veto from my parents that I didn't dare override.

A few decades later: professional and personal trials and burnout.

So: personal reconstruction, rethinking and retraining ... Neuro Linguistic Programming first, then hypnosis training developed by a hypnotherapist, but I was looking for something else...

The magic of the universe enabled me to take the SP training with Ludovic in the summer of 2023.

So, I'm a beginner at every level, but deeply happy being able to help and plant seeds of joy and love.

Case Study

A consultant contacted me about macular oedema in her right eye and, if possible, stabilisation of her sight loss.

This person suffers from "Usher Syndrome".

 I knew nothing about this pathology, so I searched for information. I discovered that this disease causes loss of sight and hearing loss and has a genetic origin.

During the session, I naturally asked the SC if there was anything that can be done about genetics, heredity, and to my great surprise the answer was No.

After the session, the client informed me that medical research into the genetic origin of her deafness and sight was underway.

She called me back to share the results, The SC had of course given the answer before the tests, the sight problems are not from genetic origin despite the pathology!

During the session, the patient felt as if there were pricks in her eye and the feedback after the session was that the swelling had disappeared and that her eyesight seemed to have improved.

laurence.chemin89@gmail.com

William Salama, SP Practitioner

Paris, France

In 2017, I was looking to work more on deep trances and in particular the Esdaile state.

I found the first training course with Ludovic Louissaint (absolutely not theoretical, which surprised me at first) in Paris that offered this: the "Simpson Protocol".

 I went along, a little curious about the promises the course indicated.

And it was both a game changer and a booster in my practice, as it introduced a fundamentally different component to the hypnosis I'd been practicing before.

From the day after the course and onwards, I've coached over a thousand people using SP. At least the philosophy behind SP. Namely, working with the Superconscious Mind. Whatever you want to call it, though. What I appreciate is that, obviously, no dogma or creed is imposed. Everyone has a unique relationship with SP, and that's the point.

The Superconscious soon went from mystery to self-evident! To me, it's not the subconscious as a resource and vital emotional process etc., but perhaps a non-conscious part of each of us - spiritual, higher and objective - capable of interfacing the information field with our own data - our subconscious. In fact, in my opinion the SC works on and with the subconscious. But it's not him...

SP is not a simple tool in the sense of EMDR or NLP, nor is it a " school " in the sense of Ericksonian, Elmanian, Quantum, Spiritual, Conversational, etc....

For me, it's no longer a question of obligatory deep trance, but a simple, pragmatic meta-approach that draws on our experience as practitioners and our life learnings, because it can contain within it all the tools that the use of trance has offered since the dawn of time (shamanism, mesmerism, hypnosis, effect of the psyche, etc.).

I appreciate the freedom that working with the "Higher Self" allows. It frees us from any reserves we may have and makes us better. Because we can integrate everything into our treatment, testing, backing off, searching, investigating - or not at all. We can interact and work as we wish with the patient's conscious mind - or not at all.

Working with SP opens up a wide range of possibilities and opportunities (even above all) for us as practitioners: listening, intuition and improvisation.

For we can use SP in the strict sense of the word, be loosely inspired by it, or use it minimally depending on the session. Progress is made because practicing is full of surprises, discoveries and openings.

Some testimonials, examples:

Transferring a resource or resources (or something else) that are positive, useful and appropriate from my patient in another dimension, to my patient in ours: "I am now rich in the possibility of accessing, when I feel the need, a state that helps me cope with everything that can weaken a being in all its dimensions." (A.G, 2024)

Getting rid of a phobia (in this case, about baby teeth) in one session: "Thank you very much! Just a note to tell you that as soon as I left our session, I was able to say and write baby teeth, and I managed to read a book on the subject to my children! I still don't know how I'll react on the big day, but I'm really delighted with this development, thank you very much!" (I.V, 2023)

Overcoming the fear of a benign eye operation (note: the SC helped improve symptoms, although this was not the objective!): "I've just come from my appointment, which went very well! The dryness in my eyes has improved since last time, and I didn't feel unwell during the operation" (J.G, 2024).

The restoration of unconscious activity: "So I'll see you again for a second session. Especially as, for the past two days, I've had access to my dreams again. It was so rare, even non-existent, that I'm convinced of the link with your first session" (S.W, 2023).

Self-revelation: "Session after session, and despite a certain amount of apprehension (it's not always easy to dive into oneself), I felt like a flood of life reinvesting my body and mind, giving me the strength to achieve each of my goals. A big thank you!" (Y.P, 2022).

"A fine, respectful approach to this practice ... a genuine exploration of one's inner being, hitherto little approached. He adapted his sessions to the person's experience, enabling real transformations of being and posture, a rediscovered self-confidence, and a different openness to life. Many thanks" (G.M, 2022)

William Salama   williamhypnotherapeute@gmail.com

SP Practitioner, Luxembourg

As a hypnosis practitioner, I was trained in the Simpson Protocol by Ludovic Louissaint over a year ago. I use the Protocol on a daily basis as part of my practice on a variety of support issues.

I'm delighted to share my feedback on the Simpson Protocol and the incredible value it brings to my practice and my clients. For someone like me, who has always been a fan of direct hypnosis, this is a real revelation. The Protocol's simplicity, versatility and effectiveness have transformed the way I practice hypnosis in my office, making each session more impactful and profound.

What never ceases to amaze me about the Protocol is that it effortlessly enables a direct dialogue with the deepest part of the subconscious, in a gentle yet elegant way that feels incredibly natural and empowering for my clients. They tell me they feel more in control and deeply understood, which reinforces their confidence in the process and in their own ability to overcome their challenges and enter a new phase of their lives. The Protocol's emphasis on tapping into the client's inner wisdom fits perfectly with my belief in each individual's capacity to change his or her life.

Indeed, at the heart of the Protocol lies the power of intention, and therefore of the authorization we give ourselves to connect with ourselves in order to make things happen for the better. This notion of intention is primordial and gives the Protocol its extraordinary character. One of the keys to my learning how to use the Protocol was to understand this fundamental notion, which totally opens up the field of possibilities.

In essence, the Simpson Protocol has not only enhanced my practice, but it has also deepened the partnership between me and my clients. It has brought astonishing value to my work, and I'm genuinely excited by the possibilities it continues to offer. I can't recommend him highly enough!

CONTACT INFO contact@eh-hypnose.com

SWITZERLAND & ITALY

Annamaria La Scala, SP Trainer Switzerland, Italy

What does the Superconscious Mind mean to me?

A guide, a friend, a loving presence that connects me with my whole body at all levels: physical, mental and spiritual.

It has always been there silently, or probably just communicating in a language that I couldn't completely understand or trust in the beginning. I was busy wanting to control my life, to understand, to explain, to live mostly through my conscious mind over body and spirit.

And Superconscious was there, patient, waiting, doing the best I would allow it to do, which was often little. My Conscious Mind needed to be in control and was so sure about most things.

Then came a feeling of dissatisfaction, sadness, need for something else. Intuition started to emerge, stronger with time, with feelings about other possibilities and a strong push from within to make changes. One step at the time the conscious mind started trusting those deep signs of the body, enabling the first steps toward the unknown. This allowed a new harmony to slowly develop openness, confidence, a new profound self-conscience and the beginning of communication with my deep self and the Superconscious.

Now I sense and rely on this inner Friend and Guide. Superconscious has become an important part of me and helps me recognize and accomplish what I need. I've observed positive changes occurring more and more rapidly and I deeply feel that I am becoming the person that I am supposed to be.

Yet, because part of me is rational and because as a trainer I like to support my explanations, I once asked the Superconscious during a self-hypnosis session, for an insight to help conceptualize it, and this image came to me: a bright and beautiful sun with lots of thin rays. For me the sun symbolizes the universal energy that connects all beings, and the rays represent the part within us, the inner wisdom that guides us through our positive transformations.

This is still today my personal representation about Superconscious, the rest is feelings and trust.

My experience with Self-hypnosis in SP- Annamaria La Scala

The Simpson Protocol is an open, easy, and highly effective hypnotic process, so much so that it is sometimes difficult, at first, to believe and accept its swift solutions.

As an analytical person surrounded by methodical minds, despite my initial skepticism, I explored SP and its philosophy. I worked on building trust through self-hypnosis alongside helping clients and witnessed remarkable changes for myself and others. I experienced increased self-confidence, started opening up and feeling more at ease speaking in public. Moreover, after more than 20 years of irritative chronic cough, symptoms improved noticeably.

Teaching self-hypnosis with SP became very quickly a central part of my practice to encourage the clients to acquire this new tool, to start making themselves the improvements they wanted in their lives and open up to possibilities. Sometimes the confidence came rapidly, sometimes gradually but the feedback was very encouraging and, unlike any other self-hypnosis processes I had learned in my previous trainings, this was for me, by far, the easiest, fastest and most enjoyable way of doing it. It was dynamic, interactive as I learned to directly communicate with my Superconscious Mind.

I started organizing ½ day workshops, following Ines Simpson's model, where the participants could begin working on any issue important to them and progress from there: from everyday concerns to more significant health-related challenges.

Stories emerged, like a teacher who used self-hypnosis to desensitize himself to clean up after a student threw up in class. He did what was needed without feeling any discomfort, numb to the smell.

Another story involves an advanced cancer patient who learned to work with self-hypnosis in a few sessions. Several months later she called to say that she was amazed at how well it worked, she could manage anxiety, sleep, pain issues and chemotherapy side effects. After a couple of years, she let me know that she was well and still using self-hypnosis.

Or a doctor who couldn't believe at first that by simply asking the Superconscious mind for something it would really work. One day he found himself in pain when during a blood test the nurse couldn't locate the vein to insert the needle. He then felt motivated enough to do the self-hypnosis and quickly anesthetized himself for the first time. Since then, he has been a believer!

Or another client that never had time to do self-hypnosis in her everyday life, one day several months after the training, went on a very bumpy and frightening flight. She remembered then about SP and could easily get rid of the anxiety and feel at ease for the rest of the trip.

Real stories demonstrate the potential and variety of applications. Learning and practicing self-hypnosis with SP is a journey worth taking and an investment for life. It is about curiosity, openness and trust, with the potential to make significant positive changes.

It is for me always a joy and a wonder to witness the creativity people develop to put self-hypnosis with SP to work.

Annamaria@lascala-hypnose.ch   Switzerland – Geneva

PORTUGAL
Helena Sousa, SP Trainer - Portugal

For as long as I can remember, I have been fascinated by the diversity of human personalities. Some people are shy, while others are extroverted; some are confident, while others are insecure. This myriad of personalities and behaviours has always sparked immense curiosity in me and inspired me to learn more about the human mind and how people can overcome their personal limitations.

Although I was raised to pursue a corporate career, as soon as I started working and earning my own money, I was able to explore this field. It was then that I first heard of NLP and hypnosis in a therapeutic context. In 2004, I flew to London to attend my first NLP Practitioner training course with Dr. Richard Bandler, and I was so captivated by it that I felt compelled to learn more.

I went on to complete my NLP Master Practitioner certification and then certified as a hypnotherapist through the London College of Clinical Hypnosis, which enabled me to start taking clients as a side job in 2010. I was finally able to facilitate change processes for clients seeking to live more fulfilling and meaningful lives, supporting them in overcoming their personal challenges - whether emotional, behavioural, or related to their mindset, and helping them pave the way to the life they desire.

And, over this time, I have never stopped studying, always searching for new and improved ways to help my clients achieve their goals. During the COVID-19 lockdown, I attended an online hypnosis summit where I watched Ines Simpson present SP. I felt compelled to learn it due to its simplicity and effectiveness. I was thrilled to learn that Ines was beginning to offer SP trainings online at that time, so I signed up for the first available training and soon obtained my certification.

Since then, SP has become my primary approach to facilitating change with my clients. I love its holistic nature—SP essentially covers every aspect of our human existence. My passion for it led me to join Ines and the wonderful team of SP trainers to facilitate SP trainings in Portuguese, in my country, and now I am offering them both in-person and online.

And since online sessions became so popular worldwide, this enabled me to take on more clients, both in Portuguese, and in English and I was finally able to leave my corporate job and fully dedicate myself to what I love most—guiding individuals through personal growth and change while teaching enthusiastic people to

elevate hypnosis to the next level with SP.

And why SP? The Simpson Protocol provides me with a highly effective structure for hypnosis-based change work. It's a comprehensive, adaptable approach that can address the widest range of client concerns.

I particularly appreciate that SP allows me to receive constant feedback from my clients during my sessions, eliminating any guesswork about the effectiveness of my interventions. And it's so simple. All I have to do is engage in this negotiation with my client's Superconscious mind, facilitating a collaborative process aimed at achieving the best possible result for them.

SP is equally effective for adults, adolescents, and children.

I would like to share one of my favorite stories with SP, which illustrates the simplicity and effectiveness of the process and reinforces that it can work not only for adults but also for children.

Maria, an 11-year-old girl, developed type 1 diabetes two weeks after her grandmother temporarily moved in with her family following an assault where she was beaten and robbed at home.

Two years prior, Maria's family home had also been robbed while they were out, prompting them to install an alarm system to increase their security at home.

Witnessing her grandmother's vulnerability left Maria fearful of being a victim herself of a similar attack, despite the alarm system.

Consequently, she experienced severe anxiety about being alone in her room, sleeping independently, and remained hyper-vigilant to all potential dangers around the house, ultimately resulting in her diabetes diagnosis.

Concerned for her daughter's well-being, Maria' mother sought hypnosis as a means to address her daughter's anxieties and restore her sense of safety. She contacted me, and we embarked on this therapeutic journey together.

This marked my first experience with hypnosis involving children, and Maria responded exceptionally well to the Simpson Protocol. Despite her age, she engaged with the process effortlessly, and all sessions were conducted online.

I began by establishing a strong rapport with Maria to foster trust and openness, ensuring the sessions were enjoyable and not perceived as a chore imposed by her mother. I hardly had to adapt my language while talking to her because she was mature enough to engage in an average adult conversation.

Although initially reserved, Maria gradually became more at ease and shared valuable insights about her feelings and experiences, facilitating the establishment of session goals and tailoring the protocol to her specific needs.

First, we addressed Maria's insecurities, fear of being alone, and concerns about safety at home. Then, we worked on her relationship with her father, whom she perceived as emotionally distant and not contributing to her sense of security. Additionally, we focused on boosting her self-esteem, which was affected by the changes imposed on her lifestyle following her diabetes diagnosis. She felt "different" from other kids and spent more time alone, away from her friends. Finally, we addressed her glucose blood levels, which were quite unstable at that time, requiring her mom to wake up several times during the night to take measures.

From the first session, I encouraged Maria to connect with her Superconscious mind and practice self-hypnosis daily, which proved immensely beneficial. Her mother ensured she followed through with the practice, reporting gradual improvements in Maria's well-being and ultimately in her blood glucose levels.

Following our four sessions together, Maria began going to her room by herself, slept alone, and felt completely at ease at home. She regained her confidence, her behavior returned to normal, and her mom expressed immense gratitude for our work together.

Working with Maria was a very enjoyable experience for me. Children are naturally curious, honest, and less likely to question or doubt the process compared to adults, making it easy to produce great results. You merely need to make sure the session is engaging and interesting for them, and they will easily collaborate. And create their own successful outcomes.

Helena Sousa   helena.sousa@gmail.com

Chapter 4- N. America

NOTE: Ines Simpson

I live on Vancouver Island on the West Coast of Canada. But my first teaching began at the NGH Conventions in the US.

I think my first official non-convention class was in Seattle, Washington.

But my client's work was in Nanaimo and then Parksville, Vancouver Island.

I did some small classes for SP there, and in Vancouver itself. Gradually expanding from Classes of maybe two or three people to 25 – 30.

What follows are contributions from many of the students I have taught over the years, and students of the trainers I have trained.

Let's start with my two favorite SP Trainers in the U.S – **Tim Horn** and **Greg Beckett.**

Tim Horn was actually the first person I picked to be an SP Trainer, but we never got round to making it official until quite some time later.

Tim lives with his wife in Manassas, Virginia on a big acreage with horses and dogs. Lots of horses!

He is a retired schoolteacher who I met at the NGH – and his teaching skills make him a wonderful SP Trainer

Tim Horn, SP Trainer, USA

Viginia

As we have been utilizing the Simpson Protocol for these many years, the one constant is the fact there are no limitations to the issues that can be successfully addressed.

In January of 2016, I received a call from Maura Sulivan asking for help with a diagnosis. Her doctor said that she had cancer. His prognosis was that she had three months. With that call, Maura determined that she was not willing to accept that limitation to her life or health.

I asked one simple question, "Is it all right with you if your doctor is wrong?" Here strong voice responded, "Yes." As a hypnotist, I like to say I am your neighborhood mind mechanic, but my clients are driving their own car.

Maura from the first moment determined she was not a cancer patient; she was a cancer survivor. Using a general protocol session, Maura created a positive outlook that saw everything in her life as a step toward becoming cancer free. Chemotherapy was used to identify and eliminate only cancer cells. Any negative effects from chemo were minimized. Her nurses marveled at the fact her hair remained in tack and while her energy took a hit, her recovery from these sessions astonished her doctors and other health professionals.

As her health continued to improve, her doctors and health team were amazed at the progress she made. With every positive comment, Maura silently chuckled to herself with the knowledge she was positively taking control of her health and future. The Protocol instilled in her the understanding that cancer was not congruent with the life she was living.

She had danced with cancer for long enough and it was time to change partners. Maura continued with all her doctor's orders, but her Superconscious Mind took all the treatments, all the comments, all the effort everyone gave her changing modifying and releasing them for her greatest good.

Eight months after our initial session, Maura scheduled a biopsy with her doctor to identify the nature of the small remaining growth within her body that could not otherwise be classified. Three nodules were taken and classified as NSD - No sign of disease.

In the five and a half years that have passed, Maura has up with her doctor and despite some scares remains healthy and vital.

The Simpson Protocol reminded Maura of just how powerful, resilient and in control she could be when the vagaries of life appear in her path. This is the epitome of client-based care any hypnotist should strive for.

To this day, Maura is an example of what a person can achieve when they allow and become aware of their Superconscious Mind.

And from another wonderful Client

How Tim Horn at HypnoConsult changed (maybe saved) my life.

Background

In 2019, at the tender/wise/old age of 72, I was in great shape, had a wonderful wife, a healthy lifestyle, terrific social and business relationships—all I could ask for. We had a perfect Fourth of July celebration with about 30 people, one of which apparently passed on a nasty case of strep a couple of days later. I had a bad allergic reaction to the antibiotic that was prescribed, and it took a couple of days to rectify the problem, at which point I was dealing with both pneumonia and pleurisy—not a good combination. After dealing with the extensive fluid buildup in my chest, my doctor did a follow up exam, checked my pulse and heart, and announced, "You have atrial fibrillation." I'm an old U.S. Marine jet pilot, I'm active, I routinely cut and split wood by hand, and I've never once had any issues with my heart—I'd heard the term "afib" but never knew anything about it.

After my first ever visit with a cardiologist, I learned that afib is basically the upper and lower chambers of the heart getting out of sequence/rhythm, causing an erratic heartbeat—not the steady 60 beats a minute or a healthy heart. I found out that afib is caused by a malfunctioning electrical system, where the nerves in the heart are thrown out of rhythm. I learned that I could still do whatever I wanted but that I was at increased risk of having a clot and a stroke—unsettling, to say the least, and scary. I was prescribed anticoagulant medication (Xarelto), which caused me to bruise easily and to bleed more vigorously after even minor cuts and scrapes. My afib caused me to breathe faster (pant) when getting any exercise, and to tire quickly—I wanted my heart to be fixed.

My cardiologist recommended the "Cardio Conversion" procedure, which basically is like a defibrillator—paddles would be placed on my chest, an electrical shock would be administered to stop/reset my heart muscles with the goal of restarting my heart in a normal sinus rhythm. Before I started flying airplanes in the Marine Corps, I was a computer/radar technician with a healthy loathing of having electrical shocks administered to my body—I was not looking forward to experiencing the Cardio Conversion process!

Exploring Alternatives

I signed up for the Cardio Conversion and was scheduled for the procedure in early August 2019. During the intervening days, I

wondered if my hypnotherapist could be useful in helping me deal with the stress of anticipating getting "zapped" in my chest. I've known Tim Horn for about 15 years—he was (and continues to be) a real hero for how he helped my late wife deal with unbearable pain and suffering. He has helped me to embrace techniques for invoking my superconscious mind, enabling me to deal with pain from injuries and the lingering effects of PTSD, and allowing me to recognize and welcome the benefits of my life.

When I contacted Tim about 5 days before my scheduled Cardio Conversion, he simply said, "I'll send you something later today" (July 30, 2019). Late that afternoon Tim sent me an audio file that I could play on my phone every night. The audio is about 17 minutes long—it begins with Tim's voice leading me into a relaxed interaction with my super conscious mind. After a couple of minutes, the sound of a heart beating at 60 beats per minute is superimposed over Tim's voice—the heartbeat continues for the entire audio. Tim's voice led my superconscious mind to accept "the new normal" of a steady healthy heartbeat.

The Result

After playing the audio file every night for 3 days, my heartbeat was beating normally through most of the day—I would feel my afib kicking in for an hour or so at a time. I was delighted with the changes and felt more optimistic about my upcoming Cardio Conversion procedure.

On the morning of my procedure, I was admitted to the hospital and prepped for the event. A nurse took my EKG, gave me a funny look, and sent it to my cardiologist. When he arrived, he checked my EKG then checked my heartbeat closely and said, "Mr. Crafts, you're in perfect sinus rhythm—your heartbeat is normal." I replied, "Yes, I know."

 My cardiologist asked, "What do you mean, you know? What did you do to get your heart out of afib?" I hesitated a little and said, "Basically, I just thought about it." After I explained the work I'd done with Tim Horn a few days before, the cardiologist said, "Well, we can't do a Cardio Conversion if your heart is already in good rhythm, so you may as well just go home."

About a year after avoiding the Cardio Conversion, I stopped taking the anticoagulant, which (in addition to stopping the bruising and bleeding) eliminated several side effects that made me feel lousy.

 I have been basically afib free for almost 5 years now—my doctor simply shakes his head every time he listens to my heart and says, "You're in perfect sinus rhythm, as usual—I've never known anyone who beat afib by basically thinking it away."

I still make use of Tim's techniques for invoking my superconscious mind and using the power that it brings to bear for making my life better. I have a very short list of heroes that I've known in my 77 years, and Tim is one of them.

Tim Horn   Tim@Hypnoconsult.com

Greg Beckett, SP Trainer USA

Los Angeles

Greg is a is a soul centered SP Trainer/Practitioner who assists everyday people to get "unstuck" from difficult life situations. In his work, Greg places a major emphasis on helping clients to see themselves more clearly and find effective ways to discover creative alternatives and innovative solutions to reignite hope and generate new possibilities for personal transformation.

Greg also has 25 years of experience in the entertainment industry, advertising, media research, and data sales. His knowledge of the entertainment and corporate worlds has given Greg insight into the day-to-day issues that cause stress and other related difficulties in the lives of executives, creative, and many others.

Through his open and accepting approach, Greg effectively assists clients to move through difficult moments of personal transitions associated with job or relationship changes or the releasing of old fears and historic challenges.

When I began my journey as an SP Practitioner, I invited friends and past clients to come in to experience the protocol as this would give me some good practice with Simpson Protocol.

One friend a woman in her early 50's, took me up on the offer. She had never experienced hypnosis with me though we had known each other for a good 10 years. I was actually surprised and happy she volunteered for a session.

When she arrived for her session, after a bit of a chat and catch up, we began the pre talk and moved into the session with SP. When I say that outwardly there were no signs or movement other than ideomotor responses (yes/no finger movement) – really no movement at all. It would seem like it was a very nonevent session from my outward observation. What many practitioners already know, outward appearances during a session do not always indicate what is happening internally –what is changing in the deepest of the client's being.

After she emerged from this "noneventful" session, my friend began to sob for several minutes. When she composed herself a bit I asked if she would like to share her experience or debrief with me what the tears were about. She said no, she didn't want to share and appreciated the session. This left me wondering what happened to/for her and at the same time I let it be, knowing this was her journey, though still curious.

About a year later, this same friend and I were in a car headed to an event she invited me to attend with her. I asked her if she didn't mind and since some time had passed, if she would be willing to tell me what had happened during her SP session the previous year. She said she thought we had already discussed it and said she would be happy to tell me now, what transpired. So, me with curiosity on the edge of my seat not knowing and completely unprepared of what I was about to hear, asked her, "what happened?" She very calmly said to me "Well Greg, I had a conversation with God."

 I was surprised for sure. Those were not words I expected to hear and didn't pursue it any further, knowing she would reveal in time anything else she felt I needed to know.

Greg Beckett   greg@hypnosisla.com

Claudia Dagnino, SP Trainer, Spanish and English

Claudia lives in Vancouver B.C Canada and teaches SP in Canada and Chile and other Spanish Speaking Countries

Here are some of her experiences with Clients.

TESTIMONIAL #1

From Sandra Saez (Concepcion, Chile)

First of all, I want to thank the Universe for placing Claudia in my life, she is a professional in all her words...with infinite commitment and patience that just by listening to her, you know that you are to the right place.

I am a diagnosed patient with Diabetic Neuropathy, Fibromyalgia and Severe Anxiety

When I met Claudia, my Physical being was out of control, experiencing chronic pain, nervous breakdown, using medications that would keep me immobilized...

My first sessions with Claudia were magical.

This is what O texted to Claudia the day after my first Simpson Protocol Hypnosis session: *"I am writing to tell you that last night I slept like never before. I didn't have the nightmares that I used to have every night (which used to happen three times a night), and I would wake up to go to the bathroom a thousand times! Last night I slept from 10.30 very tired, and I woke up at 7"*.

At first, I thought it was something casual, but it wasn't like that...now I no longer hate the nights. I used to experience Insomnia and nightmares, now I get to sleep and rest regularly...and my body every day wakes up healthier and less anxious. I also learned to work my Mind through Self-Hypnosis and to regain control of myself by working and listening to my Mind. I faced a particular emotional situation with a specific person and managed to unload and say everything I felt (which I previously wasn't able to do), and I managed to say what I really felt. After that event, unlike other times, my body did not hurt. Thanks to this therapy my quality of life has changed!

 I ONLY WANT TO SAY THAT I RECOMMEND IT A THOUSAND TIMES!! AND THAT EVERY EXPERIENCE YOU LIVE WILL BE MAGICAL

TESTIMONIAL # 2

(Client from Santiago, Chile)

This other testimonial is from a client of mine. This person (around 65 when I met her) suffered from Canker Sores inside her throat for as long as she can remember (5 years old) and had tried everything, traditional and alternative medicine, had a big one opened for a few months. Found significant relief after attending to my Self Hypnosis workshop, and even more happened for her after a one-on-one online session:

"Claudia, regarding the hypnosis practice of the Simpson protocol that I increasingly engage in with greater conviction due to its effectiveness, such as the reduction in size and duration of the canker sores. Concerning my personal development, I have also achieved something as important to me as expressing what I want with confidence, without fear, and setting boundaries (with a particular person) – something I had never accomplished before despite putting in all my effort. Having said that, in particular, I believe that. "

"Every day I feel better in the broadest sense of the word... for all of this, I am tremendously grateful to you. Hugs "

TESTIMONIAL # 3

"Hello everyone! I'd like to share a remarkable experience using SP. Recently, I've successfully treated severe vertigo in two clients within just one session, despite previous ineffective medication and persistent symptoms. Both cases, medically diagnosed, saw a 100% clearance of their vertigo after our session. One client received treatment online, while the other was in person. As my friend Ines wisely says, 'Ask Superconscious,' and indeed, the results speak for themselves. Remember there's no harm in asking "

TESTIMONIAL #4

Valeria Cancino (Concepción, Chile)

I would like to share my testimonial regarding Claudia Dagnino and The Simpson Protocol Hypnosis.

First, I want you to know that from a very young age, and as a result of experiencing bullying, I became an extremely self-conscious person. Later, in adolescence, I was diagnosed with severe Depression and Generalized Anxiety...something as simple as taking a bus, going shopping or to a mall, or to the gym...and even attending classes was a huge challenge.

Every time I went some place my mind was restless as if something bad was going to happen to me, my mind reminded me that I had Anxiety and Panic Attacks, which could unfold at any time I front of everybody... which would make me feel so embarrassed!!

After attending the Self-Hypnosis Workshop, which was my first Simpson Protocol session I noticed that all these issues disappeared... Now I am calm and at peace with myself. I looked at myself in the mirror and saw another person, I saw who I really am! I would like to emphasize that I practice my Self-Hypnosis on a regular basis, with discipline and responsibility, since this has become my medicine. I no longer feel tormented by Limiting Beliefs that controlled my life on autopilot.

I would like to emphasize that I practice my Self-Hypnosis on a regular basis, with discipline and responsibility, since this has become my medicine. I no longer feel tormented by Limiting Beliefs that controlled my life on autopilot.

I would like to thank Claudia and the Simpson Protocol Hypnosis for this opportunity since today I live in peace and have goals.... things I had come to believe I would never achieve.

Claudia Dagnino   cdagnino.counselling@gmail.com

Patricia (Patty) Meier, SP Practitioner

Saskatchewan, Canada

How the gift of Simpson Protocol has changed my life…

I would definitely classify myself as being on the hypno-spiritual side of the practice. I certified in NGH (National Guild of Hypnosis) training in January of 2018; in order to legitimize and fully understand the work I was presently doing in Past Life Regression with friends and family.

The opportunity to learn from Ines Simpson was presented at the NGH session; Ines would be here, in person, in my hometown. I pounced on that immediately!

At first it seemed too easy; just follow these steps and trust the Super Conscious Mind to do the work for the client. IT ACTUALLY IS THAT SIMPLE! In the six years since I began using SP, I have been blessed with children as young as eight and been able to facilitate them to find peace. I like to say I am their hypnotic tour guide, taking them to the places they need to go to do the work they need to do. I work with people of any age; regression hypnosis is my specialty however I enjoy helping all clients find peace.

The story I would like to share with you is of a teenager who suffered a terrible loss at an early age; their father passed away tragically from a drug addiction. This young person heard the sound of their father's laboured breathing that dreadful morning as they were leaving for school; the man passed before the end of the day. Seven years later and with the assistance of counselling, this teen continued to suffer from trauma, guilt, and anxiety; depression had been ruled out by the doctor and counsellor.

The issues reported by the mother during the consultation included: recurring nightmares of the day the father passed, stomach-aches, difficulty sleeping, guilt, anger, anxiety, and a lack of desire to participate in normal teenage activities; even hanging out with friends was unappealing. The desired outcome was obvious; release the guilt and have the emotion released from the tragedy during the waking and sleeping hours.

In the first session, the teenager revealed to me that it was not only during their sleeping hours that they would hear the father's laboured breathing; the sound followed them during quiet times throughout the daytime as well.

During the first session, there was initial resistance establishing Superconscious responses in the hand; after recommitting to the contract, the issue disappeared, and responses came easily. In the course of the investigation aspect of the session, I asked SC directly if the breathing was actually the father trying to connect with the client? Yes. I called in the client's team including the Heavy Hitters and asked for disconnection of the attachment. This took some time to completely clear; an assertive approach through SC, directly to the father was required telling him in no uncertain terms that visitation was not allowed. I then asked SC to ensure that the client would remain free of reattachment until they made a contact request themselves. The yes response was received.

After this first session, the teenager responded they felt lighter, rested, and that this session was GREAT... as well as really weird. A week later, the mother reached out to me to report that the teen was sleeping well, at ease, and back to their activities; both mother and teen were pleased with their SP results.

Fast forward a month, the teen is missing dad and hoping to find relief in another Simpson Protocol session. This time, we cleared away the feelings of sadness and asked SP if it would be possible to go to Divine to have a visitation with the father? The yes response was followed by a beautiful golden orb coming forward, accompanied by clear and strong feelings of love, and overwhelming peace.

Below is the review the mother left on Google.

Patricia is an amazing, beautiful soul. I have taken my teenager to her for healing, and they have definitely shown progress in just two sessions. Thank you for the time you have spent with them.

I thoroughly trust the Simpson Protocol to find the root cause of any issue and to help any aged client find peace.

Thank you, Ines, for bringing this amazing modality forward for the world to enjoy!

Patricia (Patty) Meier   SparksOfHealing.ca

Yasmin Udwadia, SP Practitioner

Vancouver B. C

Glimpses of The Superconscious Mind

I had heard about this technique called The Simpson Protocol back in 2018 and had been following it for a while. As a hypnotherapist with a regression-based practice, I already had the knowing and the faith that the client's mind always knows what is best for them and how best they can heal. The underlying philosophy of SP, therefore really resonated with me. After training with Ines, I started to use SP for almost all my sessions and over the years it has evolved into the most amazing, flexible and client-centred approach I know. For the hypnotherapist, it offers a lighter, very holistic way of addressing the client's issues with a lot of extra benefits for the client along the way. (SP addresses not only what we know is the issue, but also what we don't know about, always working for the client's best outcome). For the client, it offers a wonderful way to go within, to heal, to resolve issues without necessarily going back to traumatic events, and to start a self-hypnosis practice which can take the client as far as they need to or want to go.

To understand how the Superconscious mind works in a Simpson Protocol session, let us first try to frame as best as we can, what the term "Superconscious" refers to. The Superconscious mind, a concept often associated with hypnosis and other forms of altered states of consciousness, refers to a level of awareness beyond the conscious and subconscious mind. Some may refer to it as the higher self, higher consciousness, or collective unconscious. Simply put, it refers to the HIGHEST part of our (individual) consciousness, which is also part of the universal consciousness.

This consciousness, by whatever name you may call it, is all-knowing, all-encompassing, all-powerful, a creative and wise force that has the unique ability to transform and heal.

When we connect and work with the Superconscious mind in a session, both client and hypnotherapist must let go of all assumptions, pre-conceived notions, or diagnosis and allow the Superconscious mind to bring up whatever is necessary for healing the client's issue.

When we can trust and let go, we open ourselves to healing, transformation and results that are often way more than we could have hoped for, as healing happens on multiple levels.

In a Simpson Protocol session, clients usually experience all or some of the following:

- **A sense of expanded awareness and connection to something greater than themselves:**
  The Superconscious mind is thought to integrate individual consciousness with universal consciousness. It is the aspect of our being that transcends our individual ego-self and connects us to the interconnected web of all life and all creation.
- **Healing and transformation of the issue:**
  By engaging the Superconscious mind, resolution of an issue, (releasing negative patterns or releasing past trauma affecting the client), is deep and lasting. If the client needs to know something with their conscious mind, they will receive that understanding. If they do not need to know, the work is done for them by the higher mind easily and effortlessly.
- **Access to Higher Wisdom, Creativity and Insights:**

In a Simpson Protocol session, the hypnotherapist establishes communication with the client's Superconscious mind. This may involve asking questions, seeking guidance, or exploring issues at a deeper level than what is accessible through the conscious or subconscious mind alone. Within the Superconscious mind, there is thought to be a reservoir of higher wisdom, insights, and knowledge that individuals can access through practices such as meditation, prayer, hypnosis, or deep introspection. This wisdom is often considered to be innate and universally available to those who seek it.

- **Connection to Spiritual Realms:**
  While the concept of the Superconscious mind can vary greatly depending on cultural, religious, and philosophical perspectives, many belief systems find that the Superconscious mind is connected to spiritual realms, divine consciousness, or higher dimensions of existence. It is seen as a source of spiritual guidance, inspiration, enlightenment and deep unconditional love.

It's important to note that the concept of the Superconscious mind and its role in hypnosis is subjective and open to interpretation.

As I began to work with the Simpson Protocol more and more, I have learned to trust the Superconscious mind completely. I now use SP as a framework to do almost everything. In my experience, it makes every technique better. It's an amazing protocol. It's like having this big, beautiful, brilliant energy right at hand to help us as facilitators with everything that we do for our clients. Here are a few glimpses of the Superconscious in action.

Grief and Sadness.
Mary, a 65 year old artist, contacted me as she had these feelings of intense grief and sadness that did not make sense to her, that

felt disproportionate to her life. She was also facing chronic health issues and wanted to feel physically and emotionally clear once again. During her first session, we began with soul work, progressing to clearing from the time in the womb and then into the present time.

As we were clearing some external negative energies that were impacting Mary, I asked the Superconscious mind to check if there were any more and it revealed another energy she had picked up when she was eight years old which had caused her to feel scared. I then asked if the SC could release this energy from Mary, returning it to wherever it needed to go.

Barely were the words out of my mouth, there was a flash of light that lit up her entire space, filling up my computer screen (it was an online session). I was silent while I waited for the SC to let me know the process was complete. In a SP session when we do not want the client's conscious mind to get involved, we often ask telepathic questions to the Superconscious mind. So, I telepathically asked her higher mind, "Superconscious, was that you beaming the light on the screen?" The answer was an immediate yes, with her "yes" finger responding.

The light lasted for a few minutes before it gently faded away. We completed the session and as we were doing a quick debrief, Mary reported that during the release of the energy from the eight year-old, in her inner vision, she too saw a big bright flash of light that lit her up inside. This was an amazing experience for both Mary and myself, both client and therapist; and validation that there exists this amazing consciousness beyond us, that can heal, guide, release, reprogram or do whatever is needed for our highest good. More importantly, Mary reported feeling much lighter and received great relief after just one session with the grief and sadness considerably reduced.

Anxiety and life purpose

Henry is a twenty-two-year-old man who was looking for a way to release his anxiety and often felt lost and without direction. He had suffered some childhood trauma with his parents' divorce, being bullied and having abusive schoolteachers.

In his first session, we set up the finger responses, proceeded with the soul work, and other childhood work. I then instructed the Superconscious mind to bring up whatever it wanted to one by one. Halfway through the session, as we were working through the issues, I asked Henry to tell me what he was feeling. (Note: the SC mind may bring up negative feelings for release, but sometimes also brings up positive feelings for the client). Eyes still closed, Henry reported seeing and feeling a big white pulsing, positive energy in his inner space. I asked his Superconscious to do whatever it needed to for Henry with this energy and to also allow him to know what was being done.

Henry reported: "It's filling me up inside and it's a part of me." At the very moment he said those words, there was a brilliant flash of light that lit up his entire room, and this was caught on video. Like a floodlight lasting for a few seconds, the light then went off.

Nothing had physically moved or changed in his space at that time. When we wrapped up the session, I showed him the video and he was amazed, as that is exactly what he was sensing and feeling at the same moment. He said he felt this brilliant, big, beautiful light, filling up his entire physical body and his inner space. For Henry, who had a healthy amount of skepticism before the session, this experience confirmed to him that something unique was taking place, even though he could not fully understand this. His anxiety reduced significantly after this first session.

Henry says: *"I came into the session with an open mind but also open to an idea that nothing major might occur. When I was under hypnosis, I felt relaxed and in a trance. Soon I started seeing visions and images. I saw light and I had a sensation of travelling through space. It was a profound experience. For a few days after I felt very light, happy and connected to something greater. The feeling started fading away after some time and I was reminded that this work needs to be continued daily. Meditation is a big part of it, as well as the self-hypnosis exercise that Yasmin taught me. In the months following the session I felt like I have ventured on a new path of learning and spirituality. I feel like I'm making progress in my quest to find purpose in life.*
The video that Yasmin showed me afterwards of my session and the flash of light was a powerful confirmation that there are greater powers at work than we can understand".

Superconscious does it alone

Peter is a very trusting client with a deep meditative practice. After his very first session, the Superconscious just took over. It took me a bit of digging to find out what was going on. Each time I asked if the Superconscious could do a specific task, clear an issue, or resolve something… his fingers would respond with a "no". I then asked the Superconscious if it just wanted to resolve the issue on its own, and I got a "yes" response. So, no more questions were needed, no directions given, no script was followed. The work was done in a few seconds or minutes. Every session was unique and brilliant, with his Superconscious mind doing whatever was needed. Peter has resolved anxiety, workplace dynamics, released creative blocks and connected to his guides in deep states of hypnosis, all effortlessly by using SP. Further, he was given a symbol to use in self-hypnosis, to bring his blood pressure down, which he uses everyday for the best outcome.

Agoraphobia and extra benefits

Millie is a 55 year old woman who developed panic attacks and agoraphobia (fear of public spaces and crowds) following a traumatic event. She was unable to leave her house when she first reached out to me. Session by session she improved and after five sessions the agoraphobia was resolved, panic attacks gone, and she was able to live and function normally. Along the way, she reported that she had successfully and easily given up smoking after ten years, with no withdrawal symptoms, no longer feeling the urge to smoke.

Millie writes: *"At the end of 2019, my life took an unexpected turn. Without any apparent cause, I woke up one day paralyzed by fear. Simple tasks triggered panic, and my comfort zone shrank to just my apartment. I learned I had developed Agoraphobia. Desperate for a solution, I tried various therapies and coping mechanisms, but nothing worked. A friend suggested hypnotherapy, and my hypnotherapist recommended the Simpson Protocol. Gradually, my world expanded—I could go downstairs, do laundry, and even stand outside. By the fifth session, I was no longer trapped by the fear of being in a vehicle. I was able to overcome Agoraphobia I had lived with for two years and it only took five sessions! Since 2021, I live without boundaries, thanks to the Simpson Protocol, which has become my daily therapy. The Simpsons protocol is like a cheat code for your brain and body, it expedites the healing process in ways you cannot imagine. It truly works if you allow yourself to fully incorporate the process".*

Spiritual Session

Priya is a 60-year-old woman, a student of Eastern philosophy and has been working on herself, having resolved many issues in her life. She wanted to experience an SP session and see what her Superconscious would bring up for healing. We began our session and after the basic soul and foundation work was done, there was no issue to be resolved. However, the Superconscious connected her to her guide and she proceeded to receive a long message, related to her spiritual growth and how she could best achieve it. She later told me it was exactly what she needed to receive in the moment.

The ways in which SP can be used are limited only by our imagination. If we understand the philosophy of SP- to trust in the Superconscious mind, to let go and allow it to do the work, to understand that IT knows us way better than we know ourselves and knows exactly what we need, then our issues can be effortlessly resolved. Further, positive patterns and behaviours can be established to replace the old, leading to lasting change. We may also deepen our spiritual connection or gain a new sense of expanded consciousness and a feeling of interconnectedness with all around us. I feel truly blessed to have learnt this amazing technique that is a humble reminder of how little we humans truly know.

Yasmin R. Udwadia

Email: yasmin@purpleflamehypnotherapy.ca

Website: www.purpleflamehypnotherapy.ca

Deepali Agarwal, SP Practitioner.

Tennessee.

As a hypnotherapist, I have embarked on a deeply rewarding journey dedicated to facilitating profound transformation and healing in the lives of those I serve. Rooted in a passion for holistic wellness and spiritual exploration, my path as a hypnotherapist has been shaped by a commitment to address the underlying causes of emotional, psychological, and spiritual imbalances through the gentle art of spiritual hypnotherapy, using the Simpson Protocol.

My decision to pursue the path of spiritual hypnotherapy was deeply influenced by my experiences as a healthcare provider within conventional medical settings. While conventional medicine offers invaluable treatments and interventions for physical ailments, it often focuses primarily on addressing symptoms rather than underlying root causes.

My odyssey commenced years ago when I embarked on a quest, enrolling at the University of Metaphysical Sciences. Here, amidst the vast expanse of existential inquiries, I found myself drawn to the profound realms of hypnosis, spiritual transformation, and the extraordinary healing capacities of the mind.

Simpson Protocol resonated with me deeply, offering a holistic framework for addressing the root causes of issues and facilitating deep healing on multiple levels. It serves as a complementary and holistic addition to conventional treatments, addressing the root causes of illness and promoting overall well-being. Integrating SP into medical care can enhance patient outcomes, empower individuals to actively participate in their healing process and foster a more comprehensive approach to health and wellness.

As a result, The White Lotus was born to provide Simpson Protocol hypnotherapy services, taking traditional hypnotherapy to the quantum level and beyond. As a hypnotherapist, I am humbled and honored to witness the profound transformations that unfold as individuals reclaim their power, embrace their truth, and step into the radiant light of their highest selves.

The ensuing case studies illustrate real-life instances where individuals harnessed the power of spiritual hypnosis to reclaim ownership of their lives.

CASE STUDIES

Case Study 1: Embracing Wholeness: Self-Acceptance and Improved Self-Image with Spiritual Hypnosis

Introduction:
In the labyrinth of self-doubt and emotional turmoil, the journey towards self-acceptance and inner peace can be arduous. This case study delves into the transformative experience of Sarah, who found solace, empowerment, and renewed vitality through the practice of spiritual hypnosis.

Background:
Sarah, a successful corporate executive, grappled with deep-seated insecurities, a negative self-image, and cravings for unhealthy foods.
Despite outward success, she harbored a sense of dissatisfaction, trapped in a cycle of self-sabotage and emotional turmoil.

The Journey:
In the sacred space of spiritual hypnosis, Sarah embarked on a voyage into the depths of her subconscious mind and beyond, unraveling the intricate layers of self-limiting beliefs, emotional

wounds, and ingrained patterns that hindered her path to self-acceptance and well-being. She confronted the shadows of her past, embracing forgiveness, compassion, and self-acceptance. With each session, Sarah cultivated a newfound sense of inner peace, reclaiming her inherent worth and embracing the beauty of her authentic self.

Outcome:
As Sarah's journey of self-discovery and healing unfolded, she learned to challenge the negative self-talk and distorted perceptions that had plagued her for years, replacing them with affirmations of love, strength, and empowerment. She emerged from the cocoon of self-doubt and insecurity as an embodiment of self-acceptance, resilience, and inner peace. Armed with newfound clarity and empowerment, she embraced life with renewed vitality and purpose.

Case Study 2: Embracing Freedom: Overcoming Postpartum Anxiety and Fear of Public Spaces with Spiritual Hypnosis

Introduction:
In the delicate period of postpartum adjustment, new mothers often grapple with a myriad of emotions, including anxiety and fear. This case study delves into the transformative journey of Stephanie, who found solace, empowerment, and newfound freedom through spiritual hypnosis as she confronted her fear of getting sick in public places after the birth of her child.

Background:
Stephanie, a first-time mother, found herself consumed by overwhelming anxiety and fear following the birth of her baby. The prospect of venturing into public spaces filled her with dread, as she harbored deep-seated fears of contracting illnesses and endangering her infant's health. The once-simple act of stepping

outside had become fraught with apprehension, threatening to suffocate her newfound joy of motherhood.

The Journey:
Seeking refuge from the shackles of fear and anxiety, Stephanie turned to spiritual hypnosis as a gentle yet powerful tool for transformation. In the sanctuary of hypnosis, Stephanie surrendered to the depths of her mind, peeling away the layers of fear and anxiety that had taken root within her psyche. She traversed the landscape of her inner world, uncovering the root causes and hidden triggers of her postpartum fears. With spiritual guidance and wisdom, Stephanie reconnected with her innate capacity for resilience, strength, and self-healing. She cultivated a deep sense of trust in her body's natural ability to protect and nurture her child, releasing the grip of fear that had held her captive for so long.

Outcome:
As Stephanie continued her journey of self-discovery and healing, she experienced a profound shift in her relationship with fear and anxiety. Armed with newfound awareness and inner strength, she ventured forth into the world with confidence and grace, liberated from the constraints of her postpartum fears. Whether it was navigating the aisles of the grocery store, dining out at restaurants, or attending social events, she embraced the boundless possibilities of life, knowing that she held the power to create her own reality.

Case Study 3: Awakening to Life: Overcoming Suicidal Thoughts and Emotional Turmoil with Spiritual Hypnosis.

Introduction:
Within the depths of emotional despair, at times some relationships often leave individuals feeling trapped, powerless, and emotionally drained. People in these situations often grapple with the overwhelming burden of suicidal thoughts and emotional turmoil. This case study explores the transformative journey of Lisa, who found solace, healing, and empowerment through spiritual hypnosis amidst the shadows of despair.

Background:
Lisa, a successful marketing executive, sought guidance to navigate her tumultuous relationship with a loved one.
She felt suffocated by the weight of unresolved conflicts and the constant erosion of her self-esteem. The resulting emotional emptiness left her teetering on the brink of despair, plagued by debilitating suicidal thoughts and a pervasive sense of hopelessness.

The Journey:
Desperate for change, Lisa turned to spiritual hypnosis as a holistic approach to unravel the emotional complexities entwined in her relationship and to reclaim her inner peace and emotional sovereignty.
In the sacred space of connection with the Super Conscious Mind, the place of all knowing, Lisa embarked on a transformative journey to confront her deepest fears, unravel the roots of her emotional anguish, and awaken to the infinite reservoirs of inner strength and resilience within her. She delved into the recesses of her inner depths, shedding the layers of self-doubt, shame, and despair that imprisoned her spirit. She learned to disentangle

herself from emotional manipulation and regain control over her thoughts and emotions.

With each session, she cultivated a sanctuary of inner peace and serenity, nurturing the seeds of self-love, self-compassion, and self-worth that had long lain dormant within her soul.

Outcome:

As Lisa continued her journey of self-discovery and healing, she experienced a profound shift in her relationship dynamic with her loved one. Armed with newfound clarity and emotional resilience, she confronted the underlying issues plaguing their relationship with courage and grace. While the journey was not without its challenges, Lisa emerged from the shadows of emotional turmoil and despair as a radiant embodiment of resilience, grace, and self-empowerment.

CONCLUSION

The journeys shared here epitomize the transformative potential of spiritual hypnosis in transcending fear, anxiety, and self-limiting beliefs. Through the gentle guidance of SP Hypnosis, individuals can reclaim their sense of agency, inner peace, and freedom, unlocking the door to a life of joy, fulfillment, and spiritual renewal. As these stories illustrate, the path to healing begins within, illuminated by the sacred light of self-discovery and empowerment.

Deepali Agarwal: <u>deepalihypnosis@gmail.com</u>

Contact info: <u>www.whitelotuswisdom.com</u>

Fay Kelly SP Practitioner

Texas

The Story of John

A 37-year-old highly functioning autistic man move from California to Texas and within a year lost his father and only guardian. He knew me from California and his father arranged for him to see me for difficulties with the transition to Texas.

After the father passed the family had me see him (I will call him John even though it's not his real name) to help them cope with the passing of his father. In some autistic people there is a characteristic of very obsessive behavior. Using regular hypnotherapy techniques, I worked with John to help him reduce his stalking behavior. John had some relief from the anxiety, grief and stalking behavior and being forced to live in a group home as there was no one to care for him. I wasn't satisfied with his improvement using my 25 years of experience and training in many hypnosis protocols and decided to contact a guardian back in California about doing an SP session to improve John's functioning in the different areas he was having problems with. John also was prone to violent sudden attacks and with a very anticipated trip to Disney World, there was much concern from family members about whether he could tolerate the travel, long lines etc. without outbursts or violence.

I was stunned and happily surprised to see how quickly John was able to go into the state of hypnosis that is necessary for an SP session especially with his autistic challenges.

I focused one session entirely on obsessive behavior of a newscaster in California and a few other obsessive habits.

The other session was to see if his violent outbursts could be controlled or modified. In both sessions there was a lot of work being performed on the functioning of his brain and also genetics and family.

I am pleased to report that both his obsessive behavior regarding certain people was diminished, and he ceased constantly obsessing over them.

Regarding the violent outbursts, he was able to go to Disney World, changed living environments in Texas and subsequently move back

to California into a new housing environment with NO VIOLENT BEHAVIOR! To this day his improvement in dealing with issues remains strong.

To personally experience how the Simpson Protocol can dramatically change people with conditions that are thought of as untreatable by current knowledge speaks to the importance of this modality be investigated and utilized worldwide. From my own personal experience…. I believe what happened with John was nothing short of a miracle!

Fay Kelly   fayakelly@yahoo.com

Kristyn Baker, SP Practitioner

Minnesota

Kristyn Baker is a spiritual and energy healer who utilizes her training as an Emotion Code Practitioner, a Simpson Protocol Practitioner and her intuitive gifts to help clients clear past emotions and open to their own true light and inspiration.

I was first introduced to Simpson Protocol by a friend and confidant of mine who gifted me my first SP session with Greg Beckett who is an SP Practitioner and SP Trainer. All she asked of me was that I went in without any preconceived ideas of what the session would be. This was a bit challenging for me as the only exposure to hypnosis I'd had was watching people doing things on stage that was seemingly just given to them by suggestion but most likely something that they'd regret later. But I did my best.

I was both nervous as well as a bit excited at that initial session with Greg. The conversation was light and casual and within just a few minutes, I felt as though I was talking to a friend.

Greg asked me to identify what I'd like to work on and for me, I had both a physical "want" as well as an emotional one. I'd just finished Physio on my back and although it had helped a great deal, I still had a "2" on a scale of "10" level of pain that just seemed to hang on. I also was considering a change in career, which, at the time, seemed like a big leap. I had worked with my husband for the past 15 years originally in our own private practice, but for the past five years, within a health care system. I had a great desire to try my hand selling real estate but felt anxious about leaving something that I felt that I knew like the back of my hand, to something completely unknown. I didn't know how to identify what it was in this regard that I wanted to work on emotionally but shared with

130

Greg that I'd like to remove any obstacles of fear that stood in my way. With that, we got to work.

I recall that as we moved into the session, my conscious mind just would not let go. I listened to the words and despite my promise to do otherwise, I had an expectation that within a minute or two, I'd simply check out in the session. I recall counting down from 100, wondering if I might be the one person that this just wouldn't work for.

As the session continued, my conscious mind continued to hang on, answering the questions that Greg posed with a knowing "yes" of "no".

 When I'd about given up, it was then that I gave in.

Greg asked if I wanted to meet with Council. Sounding like something along the lines of the principal's office, my head said a resounding "no" while my "yes" finger indicated that I did. "What?" I asked. What was happening?

 I recall seeing beautiful spikes of energy and feeling a sense of incredible love and acceptance.

 I was asked a question by these united beings of consciousness and that question was if I still chose to continue on with my original plan for bringing healing to the world – a plan that I'd had as a spirit light before coming here in physical form. I felt a resounding yes fill me. I also felt such an incredible sense of being a part of a bigger All; a feeling that felt both eerily familiar as well as brought me such great comfort.

With that, a light messenger came for me and walked me from this great hall of light. On the walk back, the guide told me that he wanted to show me something before returning me to conscious form. With that, we stood before a beautiful patina double door. The guide opened the door, and we walked in to see a workshop of sort.

 The guide took my hand and told me that we were in the Universal creative workshop.

He pointed out Leonardo Da Vinci in one corner who intently chiseled the front piece of a block of clay. I heard music and looked opposite to another man furiously scribbling on a tablet. "Mozart" he said to me. I felt an incredible sense of awe.

My guide then told me that creating life and beauty is this simple. You simply just start to create whatever you want, whatever you envision but first you must connect to your own higher self. With that, it begins.

I was fascinated as I watched a workshop full of what looked just like ordinary people creating extraordinary things. It was then time to go and shortly thereafter, my session ended.

After Greg allowed me to emerge- he showed me how to use SP Self Hypnosis. Giving me the tools to do my own self-hypnosis.

Greg asked if I had any comments on the session and I told him about my session journey.

I told him that I felt that until the moment that my head said "no,' while my finger said "yes," I was really skeptical as to if anything was really happening to me. He laughed and told me that that was completely normal.

He then asked if I felt any difference with my lower back. I straightened my shoulders and turned my hip a bit, but the truth was, my back felt about the same. He assured me that that was just fine and that whatever was to happen, did happen. He also told me that sometimes there are changes that the session just sets in motion and often times, following a session, there is additional information, movement, understandings and healings.

That night I went to bed earlier than normal because I wanted to spend some time practicing the self-hypnosis tools that Greg had shown me.

I lay on my back, and I envisioned my lower back and hip being completely healed. With that, I fell asleep.

About three in the morning, I woke up with a prickly feeling in my lower back and leg. I lay there just allowing the feeling to move through. After about thirty minutes, the feeling subsided and I drifted back to sleep.

 Three hours after that, my alarm went off and I climbed out of bed

and headed downstairs to start the coffee. As I bent down to get water out of the water cooler, it occurred to me that I wasn't feeling any kind of discomfort whatsoever in my lower back/leg. I lifted my leg up and down a few times and then back and forth. Nothing. My right side felt exactly the same as my left side. I had zero pain! Wow, I thought. This really worked. I was excited and amazed all at the same time.

 It was then that I knew that I wanted to include Simpson Protocol training in my near future. I wasn't sure how that would work out, but I just intended that it would.

The story didn't even stop there. Two weeks or so later, my husband came home to tell me that he had just met with the hospital administration and for no known reason, they let him know that they had decided to increase his base salary, exactly the amount of the salary that I would leave behind in making my career change. This came out of nowhere and was completely unexpected, but I knew as soon as I heard the words, that the Universe was playing a hand in making my "leap of faith" an easy transition.

The Simpson Protocol is such an amazing tool. I tell my own clients today; it's about working through whatever is holding you back in therapy. The only difference is that it happens in an instant. All it takes is connecting, or reconnecting, to your Superconscious mind.

Kristyn Baker   kristynbaker1@yahoo.com

Chapter 5- UK and LEBANON

NOTE Ines Simpson:

I had been invited by Karl Smith of the UK Hypnosis Academy to present SP next time I was going through the UK – which was often as I was going back and forth to Europe to expand SP there.

It was to that time It was one of my biggest classes – until I went to Brazil – that was something else!

At that first class was a lovely person called Honey Lansdowne – and over tine we became strong friends.

Here's Honey…

Honey Lansdowne, SP Trainer UK and India

My story with The Simpson Protocol began in 2016 when I attended SP training with Ines Simpson in London, UK. I was already a hypnotherapist and NLP Master practitioner with a therapy practice by the sea. I had a rapidly growing business focused on helping people understand themselves better and develop their confidence and self-esteem and I also specialised in anxiety and depression.

Clients would often cry and although I had been in the therapeutic coaching space for over a decade by then and been on a lot of hypnosis courses (!), I hadn't experienced deep hypnosis myself. During the SP training I experienced a profound deep state hypnosis and truly connected to Superconscious, this connection changed my relationship with myself and my clients.

After the training, I began a regular self-hypnosis practice, using SP to connect with myself at a very deep level, the kind of self-connection that I had always been looking for.

With Superconscious and guidance to support me, I felt safe and more empowered than I ever had. I was able to heal physically (I went to the gym a lot and often had aches and pains and when I had minor surgery in 2018, they couldn't believe I used a deep hypnotic state instead of injections!), mentally (I'd always been into creating high performance states from my coaching and NLP experience but this added a further dimension), emotionally (I found myself healing things all the way back to childhood, 2 years old to be exact!).

In general, I found it easier to let things go, soften the emotional edges and find balance), but my far, my greatest growth area was spiritually. I found a new level of spirituality which allowed me to explore myself and the world around me safely and gently, without fear. I have been intuitively connected since I was 10 years old when I was not alone in my nan's garden when making mud pies. I didn't fully embrace it or know who to talk to about it so I 'avoided' it (as much as I could anyway!) mostly.

I jumped further into intuition when I trained in reiki and had some interesting experiences while working with people with reiki but again, I didn't really understand the true purpose of why this intuition had found me. As an intuitively connected, logically minded person, SP is perfect for me as it puts me in control of my own hypnotic state, processing and connections whilst allowing me to unconsciously explore, connect, release and optimise everything, whether working on myself or with others.

Since my SP training, I have used SP a lot with my clients regardless of their issue.

Over the years, I've specialised in matters close to my heart; anxiety and depression, addictions (smoking, vaping, sugar), weight loss, chronic fatigue, teens, childhood issues and inner child healing, trauma healing, confidence, self-esteem. I've always enabled self-discovery, because I believe that the more you know yourself and the more self-connected you are, the more confident and resilient you are.

I am not sharing this to say look at me, or me, me, me, I'm writing about my own experience as it's the truest way I can describe what SP is and how it feels.

Now onto some of the ways I use SP with my clients worldwide online and in person in UK, West Sussex & London.

Here are a couple of client stories (not real names to maintain confidentiality) that I hope will give you an insight to how SP can help.

Sarah - Trauma

Sarah wanted help with what she described as a 'deep-seated trauma stemming from childhood'. She was raised in a challenging dysfunctional family environment, where her emotional needs were not met and left her vulnerable to the abuse which took place. She was left feeling ashamed, worthless and scared, which over the years manifested as anxious thoughts and feelings and periods of depression.

Sarah had three sessions of SP which helped her release the blame for what happened first and foremost from herself as she had always felt that it was 'her fault'. She was able to experience feelings of self-forgiveness and self-love for the 'first time' (her words). One thing she had always thought was 'I don't deserve this life' and she said that working with the support of Superconscious and guidance made her feel less alone and more deserving. She posted this comment after working with me 'Working with Honey and the Simpson Protocol has been life changing. I've found peace and healing in ways I never thought possible. Highly recommend'.

Treena – ADHD

Treena had always struggled with relationships with men. She's had 3 serious relationships but never really felt as supported as she wanted. She also felt disconnected from a real connection, almost as if she was 'half there' (her words). She suspected she had ADHD but had no formal diagnosis. She was a deep thinker and in her 40s, thinking about which direction her life would take and her objective was to 'feel happier just being her'.

During her 2 Simpson Protocol sessions, Treena described it feeling like she had '2 brains'. In hypnosis, her busy brain was able to take a nap, and she was able to review a 'bigger brain' from a safe distance. She described feelings of 'infinite space', and she said it was the first time she didn't think of her to do list!

By understanding that it didn't have to feel like her head/brain was full, she was able to introduce a simple self-hypnosis practice which became her 'chill pill' when she needed to escape the 'madness' of life and reset at a deep level.

Marcus - Depression

Marcus was approaching retirement. He had a successful career, marriage, children but his whole life he had had what he called 'a core of inner sadness'. He had tried all manner of things to help him feel better and some had worked to varying degrees, but the sadness always returned, like it was 'deep inside him'. He found it hard to socialise and to be his true self, as he always felt that there was 'something wrong with him'.

He described that during dark periods, he would disconnect from his family and spend a lot of time alone. He also described feeling low energy. Marcus had 3 Simpson Protocol sessions. During the first session, we spent a lot of time in the soul work area and soul integration. As I observed Marcus at the end of the session, I noticed he looked brighter in complexion, and he explained that he had felt a great release. He seemed surprised, which is not unusual for client's experiencing SP!

In the second session, he explained how he had had a good week and felt more 'engaged in life'. In the second and third sessions we worked on more experiences that had caused or affected the issue he was experiencing. We also built up his ability to go into self-hypnosis with triggers that had been set, that enabled him to go back into hypnosis himself easily in the future. Humans are fluid and the more we are able to self-connect, the more good work we can do on ourselves. Marcus described the progress he made as 'life changing' and 'freeing'.

Tom – Stop smoking.

And one last client experience I will share is Tom, a middle-aged smoker in a senior position in an engineering company. He came to stop smoking and said he was not spiritual. You don't need to be spiritual to encounter Superconscious or other aspects of Simpson Protocol. When he had finished his session and had become a nonsmoker, he described that he had seen colours all around him and felt the support of Superconscious and guidance to support him, not only in his stop smoking journey, but also at work and in

life. He was very surprised by this but went with it anyway. The ideal client for a Simpson Protocol session!

Here's a poem I wrote about SP.

How glad I was to find SP,

On my journey of self-discovery.

Hypnosis that is client led,

No need to listen to what is said.

Suitable for any issue, any age, anyone,

Discovering Superconscious can be fun.

Feel self-love & self worth that's deep inside,

Once empowered, limiting beliefs can't hide.

Your higher self can step out of the shade,

New positive beliefs can be made.

Superconscious and guidance are there for you,

To support you in the healing you do.

Anxiety and depression feel smaller,

And self-esteem, well, that gets taller.

Addictions and baggage can leave now please,

A new life is yours to seize.

Find yourself, the true you,

And do all the things you want to do.

As the licensed trainer of Simpson Protocol for UK & India, I wanted to share a few comments from my trainees so you can get a feel for what training with me is like:

Ellie - I've enjoyed finding out about the processes and strategies behind hypnotherapy, learning about the conscious, unconscious mind and why we do what we do. What I really enjoyed the most ishow much Honey has given herself. It's just a really, really valuable experience around, you're not just learning, you are experiencing too.

Zoe - Don't hesitate, do it. Honey is really supportive and informative. She's very professional and really knows her stuff. She teaches and communicates, and she has a good sense of humour.

Hannah – Training with Honey is a really, really valuable experience, you're not just learning, you are developing yourself too.

Elaine - Honey is insightful, has her finger on the pulse of all things that are relevant for her trainees, and delivers her sessions with an obvious love for what she does.

Honey Lansdowne www.honeylansdowne.co.uk

thesimpsonprotocol.co.uk

Isi Murray, SP Practitioner.

UK

When my soul sister and best friend in the world was diagnosed with aggressive pancreatic cancer, I didn't think twice about working with friends and family. I knew exactly what Protocol I was going to trust wholeheartedly to give her the best, fighting chance of dealing with this horrendous disease on her own terms. Personally, I was devastated, but it wasn't about me. Without chemotherapy, the best guess her doctors could provide was in the region of 4 months. At diagnosis, the doctors were far from optimistic that the necessary biliary indicators, required to even consider treatment could be achieved, particularly given the timescale.

But they didn't know about Superconscious Mind.

We got to work. We began with issues around her obvious shock at the diagnosis and the often misguided, language she was hearing at the hospital. She had so much courage, but it certainly helped to clear her mind and have her focus where it needed to be. She wanted to stay as strong as possible, both physically and mentally, throughout the process, and maintain clarity. Her goal was to maximise every second of every day with friends and relatives and just simply to enjoy herself. She was a wonderful subject, completely at ease with the hypnotic process with a sense of openness and curiosity as to what could be possible. Duly researched and adapted, we introduced the Optimal Health Template. Through this, our focus turned to the numbers so that she could have the best possible chance of treatment. I made her recordings, and she learned self-hypnosis. I admired her incredible commitment to the process. Every time I called her, she made me smile, saying "Goodnight Isi. I'm off to spend some time with Superconscious".

A matter of weeks later, her numbers were almost there, and the doctors were so shocked at the drastic drop. Chemotherapy was on the table at last. I was over the moon for her but the joy, on my side, was short-lived. She had given it so much thought with that clarity that she worked so hard to achieve and decided that she did not want to go through the treatment for the limited time benefits it would give her. She decided that she wanted to live out her days to the absolute maximum. We discussed her outcome in greater detail, and I realised that it hadn't really changed. Appropriate, optimal and beneficial for her still meant the same thing - she wanted to complete her journey with the minimum of fuss, the maximum of pleasure and the least possible discomfort for her family. She didn't want to have to endure a painful, long drawn out ending to her life. She wanted to smile as long as she could. She had chosen the path she had worked towards all along. She had simply given herself an option just in case.

She booked her plane tickets to come and spend a week with me and she booked up as much of her calendar as she could with outings and meetings with friends and family, even the odd rock band! And we got back to work, keeping her outcome at the forefront of our minds and sessions together. She knew exactly what she wanted and Superconscious was there at every end and turn to help her achieve it. Chakra sessions and spiritual sessions followed, making sure she was completely at peace with her decision, the inevitability of that decision, her approach to and management of it.

We had the most fantastic time together. She was unstoppable. There were visits to the theatre to see musicals she loved, meals out even though eating wasn't the best thing for her, and walks she loved which I'm sure weren't physically easy for her. Above all, constant laughter. We didn't work with hypnosis that week - not formally anyway. After 40 years of the best friendship anyone

could want, we didn't want to discuss the inevitable face to face, and we certainly didn't want to say goodbye. Unusually for the end of March, the sun shone for the whole week. It was beautiful weather, and we didn't miss a moment of it.

On her return home her deterioration was quick, and we could no longer work online. She went back to listening to her recordings and falling asleep with Superconscious taking her to Peace, Deep and High. Within days, with an operation scheduled for the following day, she decided to go into hospice care to avoid her son having to struggle with her failing health. The hospice was some 2 hours' drive away from her home; a long way for her two adult children and grandchildren to travel regularly. When the ambulance came to collect her, she asked for a few minutes, sat on the steps of the vehicle and shared a glass of grand Marnier with her daughter and son. It was so 'her'.

She passed away that night. She didn't want to put anybody out. She didn't want her family to have to travel. She didn't want to go through the pain of surgery that couldn't save her. She wanted to do it her way. It's what she asked for and it's what Superconscious helped her get. What's more, the hospice staff said they had never seen anyone pass away so peacefully and they were amazed to note that she was smiling. I, for one, know that she would have taken herself to Peace, Deep and High…… I love you Bev x

Isi Murray imisimurray@gmail.com

Ines Simpson DUBAI

Thanks to my good friend and excellent Hypnotist Beryl Comar I was invited to teach SP classes in Dubai two or three times.

They were always interesting classes as they would always have such a range of nationalities in each class. Arab Nationalities of course, from UAE, Syria, Lebanon, Oman and so on but also French, Welsh, English, American, Indian– you name it.

I particularly remember a wonderful devout Muslim man who was so encouraging, and a beautiful woman from Oman- who after the session was shining bright!

I was then excited when Immane Soubra from Lebanon turned up in one of our Classes held over Zoom and became the SP Trainer in Arabic.

LEBANON
Immane Soubra, SP Trainer Arabic

Here is a recent story of a lady with trichotillomania (hair-pulling disorder) she started with this habit very long ago, quoting her: "I always remember myself with this habit, this is why I don't know when it started but the thing, I know is that I tried everything possible to stop it and it was impossible." after a bit of intake, we started the Simpson Protocol session, it was intense with a lot of regressions, I gave a recording to listen to it daily that will better enhance the benefits of our session together.

After 2 weeks she called, to tell me since that session, I hadn't pulled a hair, and now after 2 months, she is still free of trichotillomania.

Immane Soubra   imanensoubra@gmail.com

Chapter 6- Down Under

NEW ZEALAND and AUSTRALIA

NOTE: Ines Simpson

I wanted to visit Australia, with SP for a long time, but it took many years to connect with the right people and set up SP Trainings there.

Plus, I had a great friend there Tony Kyprios who I had met at the NGH and was excited to re-visit – and not just because he lived in the delightfully named Toowoomba!

And I met Lance Baker who helped us in Sydney and Newcastle – an amazing man.

And let's not forget the wonderful Pamela O'Leary who fortunately for me lived in tropical Cairns and came to the SP Class there.

On my second trip to Australia – I thought well why not visit New Zealand? And SP Training there was hosted by Justine Lette

Justine Lette is amazing – no need to give her an intro of how we met – she does it better than me.

Justine Lette, SP Trainer- New Zealand, Australia

New Zealand

My introduction to Simpson Protocol.

I had helped organise the first New Zealand SP training with for Ines, when the person who was going to set things up became ill and recommended me.

I said sure I would set things up – even though I had no real knowledge of what SP was or what I was in for.

As the owner of Hypnosis New Zealand, I organise many trainings and more often than not, the trainings are the same old process - but packaged in a different way.

When the class started and the concept of Superconscious was introduced, I was intrigued. I have done a lot of work with the higher-self / higher-mind but this was a little different.

I decided I would get involved and actually join in on the group practice and when it was my turn in the hot seat, I said 'why not work on spiritual enhancement!' Well with SP, be careful what you wish for.

In the session there is a part where you go back to times or events that have caused or are affecting the issue.

 Usually, you can be unaware of where that is on a conscious level, but I remember clearly being little and seeing a scary face.

Now as an adult, I realize it wasn't scary at all (just an old, wrinkled face) but must have been quite different then.

I am guessing that is when fear started around seeing things that are not 'real' as such.

In SP we do this process in a very safe and gentle way where the client doesn't need to know any more than the age and feeling, I was just in a space to have aware of more.

What astounded me was when the session finished and my eyes opened, I saw beautiful colours around people I hadn't seen before.

I was hooked!

And then towards the end of the 4-day class Ines came up to me and asked if I would like to be the New Zealand trainer for SP?

You betcha!

I absolutely love teaching SP. I have had so many experiences then with students and clients that would be considered unreal, but with the mind and being open to possibility, anything is possible.

Case Studies

There have been so many things that have happened to my students since that class – positive – eye opening things – but here's an experience of mine:

And it was in this first class, I connected with an energy, a spirit, call it what you will – that was to be called Ultra – and would unlock many aspects of SP in the future.

It was a strange a strange experience – as every time I went into trance – there are lots of practices in an SP class – I felt this presence appear and indicated it wanted to connect through me to Ines.

Now I had not really experienced the concept of channeling before – and to tell you the truth I was getting annoyed, as I wanted to follow the class, not listen to some possibly imaginary chattering.

Anyway, just to satisfy my 'imaginings', after a class one day I mentioned this connection going on to Ines.

Ines took me away from the class – put me into trance and we connected.

A very very strong energy came through – and we had an interesting discussion – well they did, as I had no knowledge of what happened – I was blanked out of the conversation.

And that happened again – except when I flew to Canada to see one of Ines classes to finish my training to be an instructor for SP – another energy came through that wanted to talk to Ines. Again, I was blank about the interaction – they say they 'crew a veil' over my understanding.

This time, I was told later, it was a strong female energy and gave some more insights in how to take SP forward.

SP is always interesting!

A horse story.

I was doing a demonstration in class on surrogacy session on an animal. Surrogacy is working with someone on behalf of someone else. This is a neat way with children, animals or people that are unable to be there.

I had a horse that had recently had surgery on its leg and then injured another while being a little silly.

I had asked that we work on the horse and the surgery wasn't mentioned.

During the surrogacy session we connect through the surrogate (the person in the chair – usually who has some connection to the animal we are working on) to the client (in this case my Horse) with permission from the superconscious.

The Client has no conscious awareness of anything going on – but with animals I think they know some things are going on.

I was working with a beautiful student who is excellent but quite analytical like myself. I find this type of person great to work with as the experience is even more mind blowing when things happen.

We went through the session connecting with the horse and asking for the best and most appropriate and beneficial things to be done – in the session to benefit the horse.

When the session ended, the student opened her eyes and said, "that horse NEVER wants to go through a surgery like that again!"

The surgery wasn't mentioned at any point but during the session, the horse gave her a very clear message that he was displeased about having to have it.

I had to laugh because it really did match his personality, and I have to say, being stalled for weeks was not fun for a 17.3hh Thoroughbred with energy.

Justine Lette   info@hypnosisnewzealand.co.nz

Hana Zawodny, SP Practitioner

New Zealand

Overcoming Driving Challenges

Meet Sally, 47, juggling life as an entrepreneur and a super mum. Picture this: she's driving, and there's that part of the motorway that freaks her out every time. She can't explain it, but it's like her body hits panic mode – heart racing, breath short – so bad once that she took herself off to the hospital because she thought she was having a heart attack.

In her first session we talked about what she believed to be the issue and then allowed her superconscious mind to take over. What we uncovered was that the issue wasn't even about driving. I utilised her superconscious to provide her with a conscious understanding of what the problem actually stemmed from and then asked for her to be filled with beautiful healing love and light. Facilitating this process helped Sally to have a new perspective around driving.

At the end of the session, Sally said she knew something had changed but she couldn't quite put her finger on what.

I invited Sally to drive the stretch of road that had been previously plaguing her before she came to her next session. She reported back that all she had now was a touch of apprehension and nerves in case the same thing happened.

In the second session I used superconscious to help Sally gather the resources and the inner support she needed to reframe driving this stretch of road to be just a road, the same as all the others she drives on.

Fast forward, and Sally's cruising along that bit of the motorway, as chill as a Sunday morning. That old fear? Gone. She's got this now.

Burnout Recovery

Laura is a 37-year-old corporate lawyer and was a textbook case of living on the edge of burnout. Her days were a blur of endless meetings, late nights, and constant pressure to perform. It seemed like the more she achieved, the more was expected of her.

Gradually Laura started feeling drained, joyless, and detached from her passions and even her relationships.

The turning point came during a major negotiation, when she realized she couldn't summon the enthusiasm or focus that her job required and was ready to quit.

In Laura's first session I used the Simpson Protocol to access the part of the mind which operates beyond our everyday

consciousness. Through the session I was guided by her superconscious to the areas that required attention and healing. This involved healing unresolved stress and reprogramming her response to workplace triggers, along with enhancing her personal boundaries and self-care routines.

As our sessions progressed Laura noticed a shift. Not only did her overwhelming feelings of exhaustion begin to subside, her perspective about work and life changed. She began to reclaim the joy in her career, remembering why she loved it so much. Outside of the office she started to introduce hobbies that she'd neglected, like painting and yoga which brought balance and happiness back into her life.

At the end of our sessions Laura reported feeling more grounded and energised than she had in years. Her recovery wasn't just about getting back to her old self, but about discovering a new, more sustainable way of living and working.

Hana Zawodny   https://www.hanazawodny.com

Rachael Hay, SP Practitioner

New Zealand

Simpson Protocol - Afterlife experience

I met Joanne in early 2023, she came to see me about the overwhelming grief that she had been feeling for her dog Bingo,

who she had had to have put down, due to his old age, and he wasn't well, and had started to suffer, and even though Joanne knew that she needed to have Bingo put down, to put him out of pain and suffering, she also felt terrible remorse for this, she said that she didn't blame herself or feel guilty, just wished she hadn't had to do it.

She also missed Bingo a lot, they had been constant companions in her life and Bingo had played a big part in her family life, spending many a day going for walks, playing with the children and generally being the family dog.

So, we agreed that it would be beneficial to do the Simpson Protocol Afterlife. After settling Joanne into trance, I went through the protocol. I asked Superconscious mind to let Joanne and Bingo connect in the most appropriate way for the session and commenced with the questions.

The questions are geared around Joanne having an experience with the passed over spirit of her dog Bingo. I let Joanne know to take as much time as she needed for the full experience, as there is no rush, the questions are geared around her taking up her time.

I could sense the emotion starting to rise in Joanne as we began the questions, she really loved and missed her dog, and the session was bringing back all her emotions around the situation.

During the session, I could at times see Joanne's expression, sometimes she looked pained, or she would smile or there would be a silent tear flowing down the side of her face. The emotion in the room was palpable.

Whenever I have a client, we connect in through Superconscious mind on a psychic level, so even though I could see the physical aspects of what Joanne was experiencing, I could also sense the emotions, sense the pain and the joy. And I could sense Bingo's essence as well.

After the session Joanne explained to me what had transpired. Bingo appeared as soon as I asked Superconscious mind to connect the two of them. She felt him lying beside her, on the left side, which he always did (this had made her cry with joy).

On one of the questions, she was shown them playing ball out in a field, with the sun shining and Bingo racing back and forth with the ball. Joanne explained to me that this was a regular activity that they shared.

Then with another question, Bingo bought Joanne his mat, which was a big part of Joanne's memories, knowing that Bingo was happily on his mat, but also there was a sadness attached with that because of Bingo when he got old and Joanne had to make that decision, him not being able to get off the mat easily made Joanne cry with the sadness of what his life had become and that she didn't want him to be in any pain.

In the last part of the session, Bingo showed Joanne a symbol, this was of a butterfly, so Bingo was letting Joanne know that whenever she saw a butterfly that this was him being around her. It also made her smile when he showed her this, because he had always chased and been fascinated by butterflies whilst alive.

So that was the first session.

I had feedback from Joanne after the session, where she said:

'I haven't been able to talk about him without crying and I went for a walk after our session and just felt so lucky and grateful and talked about him with so much happiness. Sadness was there but not to the same extent as before our session. I felt him with me and feel peace with it all'.

She also mentioned the butterflies.

'The butterfly is symbolic to rebirth after death. Beautiful. I walked out into my garden and saw 4 straight away! Tried to take a photo but they were too small to see. Thank you for today! Thank you from the bottom of my heart.'

And so, then we had a second session, and again during the session, there were the physical and emotional signals from Joanne, a slight tear here, a frown, a smile.

After Joanne emerged, she told me that she realised that she had been feeling incredibly guilty about euthanizing Bingo, but Bingo had told her during the session that he had been really unwell and had wanted to go. He knew that he needed to go, he had no quality of life and just didn't want to live in pain anymore.

Bingo also imparted to Joanne during the session how much he loved being with her and with the family and that he had a great life. He did this by showing her images in her mind, but also in feelings.

All this really released something in Joanne, and she remarked how profound it was, because even though she was feeling sad about

Bingo, she had not realised before the session how much this was bound up with her grief and her sadness about having to make

'that' decision. And that now having heard what Bingo had to say about it, she could fully understand and feel the release of all that built up emotion and turmoil. She explained this to me as tears silently flowed down her face.

She also cried with the memory of how Bingo had imparted his feelings of love to her and her family. She said that during the session, she had felt him there, leaning against her side, which is what he always did while alive. Joanne left that day still able to imagine and remember the feeling of Bingo by her side.

Rachael Hay <u>rachaelhay108@gmail.com</u>

Lilly McKenzie, SP Practitioner

New Zealand

You know that feeling you get when you sense it's the right call, the right move? That's exactly what I experienced when I stumbled upon SP. My journey with SP kicked off in 2022, sparked by a conversation with a magician-turned-hypnotherapist from New-Zealand. Maybe it was one of his tricks, but boy, was I hooked! In no time, I said 'good-bye' to the other hypnosis techniques I'd learned before and focused solely on the Simpson Protocol. The results? Twice as fast and even deeper in some cases.

The concept of the superconscious mind is a real head-scratcher. It took me a while to stop questioning it and just trust the process. When I did, the results were mind-blowing – in person, in groups, and even online! The beauty is the results hold up across the globe. I've worked on people, babies, the departed, animals, and even houses! As long as the Superconscious mind gives the "YES finger", anything is possible.

I've worked with aggressive dog behaviors, helped pregnant moms connect with their baby and conquer morning sickness fears, and aided men grappling with heavy trauma and emotional numbness. Seeing them return after a couple of sessions, radiant and with a newfound brightness in their eyes, makes you profoundly grateful for the work you do.

Clients often have no clue what's going on. They'll say things like:

- 'Why are my fingers doing their own thing?' or

- 'I could hear you, but my mind had a different answer than my fingers!'

Another remarkable thing about Simpson Protocol is that you can do self-hypnosis. I regularly work on myself to address issues and clear any heaviness. I vividly recall a time when I felt off for a few days. It was a deep-seated anger, a rage even, with some very negative thoughts about me. I decided to do a self-hypnosis session before bed to see if I could shake this feeling out.

(SC -SuperConscious)

ME: SC, does this feeling belong to me?

SC: No

ME: Did I catch this energy somewhere?

SC: Yes

ME: From a client?

SC: No

ME: Someone I know?

SC: Yes

ME: From the party last weekend?

SC: (very strong signal): YES!

ME: (thinking of someone): Is it "XY"?

SC: (big signal): Yes, yes, yes

ME: Is it a foreign energy that used "XY" to 'attack' me?

SC: YES, YES

ME: SC, can you please release this energy from me in the most appropriate and loving way?

SC: Yes

At that moment, I felt a huge weight lift off me. I became very hot and experienced hot flushes (a sign of energetic release). I was blown away, tears streaming down my cheeks, feeling calm and grateful. The anger vanished instantly.

This is just one example among many. I've resolved deep issues using this technique, both for myself and my clients. The more you trust the process and clear yourself from your own 'issues,' the better practitioner you become. I am genuinely honored and grateful for using this powerful hypnosis technique. It's become one of my missions. I apply it in individual sessions, online, and offer free group sessions.

If reading this has piqued your curiosity, try it! You'll be amazed at the power within you waiting to come up! This inner power is gentle, compassionate, and eagerly awaits your invitation to emerge.

Lilly McKenzie lilly@bodymindcare.org

Angela Freychet, SP Practitioner

Australia

I had been teaching yoga for 15 years prior to learning hypnosis. I had trained in India with the yogis diving into all aspects of yoga and meditation.

I became a past life regression hypnotherapist with the desire to explore the subconscious in more depth.

Regression therapy was efficacious to some degree, but I was looking for something else that could really get to the meat of an issue quickly and effectively.

It was through a newsletter that I first heard about SP. I went online to investigate and came upon YouTube videos of training which deeply resonated with me. I knew that I had to do it and find out more.

 The first training I did was in 2018 here in Perth, having the great privilege of studying in-person with Ines Simpson. I was totally hooked from the start. I loved Ines's playfulness. I loved the holistic aspect of SP, the simplicity of SP. I have come to appreciate how SP is constantly evolving, and everyone is encouraged to make it their own. It has changed my life in so many ways and opened my mind to the vast potential of a person. I use SP with my clients for everything - there's nothing that SP can't address.

My Session

Start here: On a personal level, my very first SP session in 2018 was incredibly profound. I had suffered anxiety for most of my life, experiencing it like a band of tightness around my diaphragm. It meant I made decisions always out of fear which held me back in so many ways.
During my very first SP training I realised, even after years of therapy, the things I thought (in my conscious mind) I'd cleaned up, were in fact, still not resolved. As the session progressed, I felt my breath change, and my whole being expand. I walked away from that session very present, but it wasn't until I was driving home that I realized that the 'familiar band of tightness' in my diaphragm was no longer there. It was an odd, eerie feeling, but similarly, very exhilarating. For many weeks afterwards I 'expected' that tightness to return, but it never did.

Sichort

Again, in one of Ines's trainings she took us into Sichort – the state of extreme body-mind relaxation whereby deep healing can occur.

I thought I'd experiment with this further at home, and before going to sleep took myself into hypnosis and intended that I move into Sichort as I slept.

I woke the next day to find that I had not moved a single muscle from the last moment I had closed my eyes. It was as if I had closed my eyes one moment, then opened them the next to find that it was daylight.

Yes, I can say that I have had this happen once or twice before, but then I woke up feeling stiff and sore from remaining in the one place. But on this occasion, I awoke with a very deep level of contentment and peace in my body and mind.

Surrogacy

In regard to clients, one of the most fascinating experiences occurred using surrogacy for children.

Surrogacy involves going into hypnosis 'on behalf' of another person or animal! There needs to be a 'permission' to access another's field of consciousness, and if that is given then we proceed with a usual protocol of questions.

My colleague (SP and I trained) often work on behalf of a client's child who is not able to verbalise or communicate or express what the issue is. One of us is the therapist asking the questions and guiding the session .The other, the surrogate, in our case, the child.

One of our child-clients aged 4 whom we had previously done work for, suddenly regressed – her mother had noticed her withdrawal and anxiety.

She was concerned that something had happened, but as the child was only 4 and she was not able to express what it was.

After my colleague took me (surrogate for the child) into hypnosis and as I was accessing that infinite field of consciousness, an image quickly flashed in my mind.

It was of our little client in a toilet block having a young boy expose himself to her!

My body-mind then felt the whole gamut of emotions that she experienced as a result of that encounter. As per a usual session, we asked all the questions to clear things up, and the feedback from her mother later that day was that she was back to her usual self again!

Another client came into my practice with deep depression and grief after her father had passed, and experienced years of unresolved issues with him.

During the session I began to notice the fingers twitching on her other hand and asked whether there was a 'part' that needed to communicate. 'YES'.

 I asked whether that part was benefiting my client by being there. 'YES'.

Was there any forgiveness work that needed to be done? 'YES'.

Anything that it needed to express to client that would be of benefit to her? 'YES'.

Can you communicate that so that the client will understand and will continue to benefit from it? 'YES'.

So, there was a long pause as that communication took place.

We moved on with the session and at the very end, as she was emerging from hypnosis and opening her eyes, the cables of my lamp in my office suddenly started shaking back and forth (no open window; no breeze!). As she witnessed the cables, she casually said, "Hi Dad...and thanks."

Angela Freychet   shunyata_71@hotmail.com

Phil Cardow, SP Practitioner

Australia

My journey with hypnosis/ hypnotherapy and healing began around 2007 when I was a young tradesman with a smoking habit. By the time I was 23 I had already been a smoker for about 8/9 years. One day in the newspaper I saw group stop smoking hypnosis sessions advertised, and for a meagre $100 investment.

 I figured why not, so I attended and an hour later walked out a nonsmoker. That easy.

Many years later, having struggled with various and often crippling anxieties surrounding money, other people, my own self-worth and more, I again enlisted the help of several hypnotherapists and realised what I had already known, that healing, and change was indeed possible, and that after going down all the usual routes (doctors, medications, counsellors) that none of these traditional approaches would ever help me.

Hypnosis had helped me realise that not only was I inadvertently responsible for every emotion, response and unpleasant behaviour that I experienced, but that I was the only one who could make these changes within myself possible.

It wasn't long after this that out of interest I attended a one-day self-hypnosis seminar which led to me enrolling in my first 'clinical hypnosis' training, then NLP, master hypnosis and master NLP and as with most of us at the start of our healer journeys, many other short courses trying to find the silver bullet as it would be. Find the one protocol that we could use with every issue, with every client.

Before learning SP in Australia with Ines's then current SP trainer IMR's and regression to cause simultaneously. The IMR's as a diagnostic tool, and the regressive techniques to do the release work. It worked well for the most part but still relied heavily on heavy energetic output that regression and chair therapy requires. Lots of tears, frequent abreactions, and after a few years of working like this day in and day out it was starting to exhaust me.

So, when I enrolled in the SP training, I honestly thought I was just doing 'another hypnosis course'. I was wrong.

 SP finally brought things together for me in a way that required MUCH less energy on me and my clients behalf's, for the most part did away with the need for my clients to actually revisit potentially nightmarish scenes, opened me up to surrogacy which has not only benefited many clients that I have worked with but allowed me to help my own son, and made dealing with the more tricky and even physical issues much easier.

It's like following a script, without ever using one. By bypassing the conscious and unconscious mind and dealing directly with the superconscious mind which is far more agreeable, makes so much more possible, and most of the time is as easy as working with the feedback that the Superconscious mind gives us, we can do away with ever having to worry about whether we, or our clients are doing it 'right'.

Thank you, Superconscious mind.

 Case Study: I've chosen a recent client (2023) as a case study of sorts. Initially Jayne (name changed) contacted me wanting to resolve two separate phobias, neither of which she could communicate to me as even talking about them triggered her so badly. Jayne was scheduled for kidney transplant surgery due to a failing kidney but couldn't attend dialysis due to her extreme phobias of both her own veins, and needles.

Even on the phone Jayne refused to tell me what she was scared of but knowing that the superconscious would know I assured her that there was a good chance I could help anyway.

On her first appointment Jayne told me that she had kidney failure and that her kidney function was currently at 14% and declining. She told me that due to the nature of the fear she was experiencing she had refused dialysis, and even blood tests though couldn't tell me why, just that she was so scared of what she had to do that she simply couldn't, she also informed me that even though she had transplant surgery booked, she had no intention of ever being able to attend and that she would likely die as a result.

After chatting for a bit Jayne finally came right out and told me she was petrified of even the thought of her own veins and blood. Terrified to think about them, talk about them, and simply couldn't face the idea that she had to undergo medical interventions that whilst would be life saving, she simply couldn't do.

I told her that that's fine, that there is a part of her that is more than capable of helping and she needn't say more.

So, our initial session was a pretty standard first SP session, nothing out of the ordinary though lots of the regressions were coming from a past life where it was made very obvious that something dreadful had happened to her. By all accounts she had had her veins and major arteries pulled out of her back in some sort of terrible tribal ritual.

Even after repeatably asking SCM to make it as comfortable for her as possible it was obvious that she was going to go through extreme abreaction, and she did. Screaming, crying uncontrollably, shaking in the chair. It was quite a long session too with most questions taking minutes or even longer to clear. Finally, nearer the two hours mark we were done (for now) and after about twenty minutes settling down Jayne was able to make it back to her car where she slept for a couple hours while she adjusted to the severe processing.

A week later when we met again Jayne was clearly deeply upset at herself and even more worried as firstly her kidney function had dropped to ten percent (down four percent in the last week) and secondly, she reported that even though last week's session seemed to go so well (albeit it being so intense for her) there had been no change in the way she felt.

I was patient knowing that sometimes serious issues can take time and often multiple sessions to resolve and as we spoke, I noticed that Jayne was now talking, openly almost about how bad her fear of needles was, but how she couldn't get her blood work done, was still refusing dialysis, and there was no way she could attend her transplant surgery.

Noticing that she was talking about what was clearly a different issue I casually asked how she felt about her veins and her blood which caused her to stop mid-sentence. She realised that she had not even mentioned them, not once, and to her bewilderment she looked at her wrists, her arms, pinched and pulled here and there and then started crying with relief as she realised that she could think and talk about them without any reaction whatsoever. Even after being a part of thousands of hypnosis sessions, by this point the change was phenomenal even by my own expectations. Such an intense and deep-rooted past life phobia completely cleared in a single session. I guess the abreactions were worth it.

Our second session together was to address the needle phobia, which was the main reason why Jayne had refused medical treatment, and it went much the same as the first. Highly emotional, heavy processing, lots of tears and physical abreactions which according to SCM was as comfortable as was possible at that time.

The outcome was much the same, needle phobia completely cleared in a single (albeit harrowing) session.

Jayne came back to my office the next week (she had paid for three sessions upfront) and it soon became clear that the breakthrough she got was much more profound than she (or I) had expected. Many other parts of her life had changed, drastically, and seemingly overnight.

We spoke for a while and I kept checking in to see if there was anything else she wanted to work on while she was there, she said no, she was at peace so I brought up the idea that maybe we should do some more work together and see what can be done about healing her kidney, I explained that physical illness's often have emotional or traumatic root causes. Jayne was very excited by the idea, so booked more sessions which went very well.

Nothing too outlandish or exciting, none (or very little) of the reactions she was experiencing in her first couple of sessions, but they were certainly emotional.

Once again, we found the root cause in a past life, I think the same one that caused the initial phobia we worked on, but for the most part they were standard second sessions with bits borrowed from the health and spiritual protocols.

We did two sessions two to three weeks apart and her kidney function, which was as low as ten percent when I first met her, was now up to 36% and climbing. Superconscious said it had done all it could for now and to allow another few weeks before we did more work.

About a month later we met again, and Janye reported her kidney function had gone up to almost fifty percent which I, and she thought was incredible. We completed her third session working on her kidney and a week later she emailed me to say it was still improving, she was having blood tests without issue and that she had cancelled her transplant surgery.

An absolutely incredible success story and testament to the power of working content free and just allowing the superconscious mind to do what the superconscious does.

I heard from Jayne once more several months later and she reported that her kidney function was now sixty something percent, she left a glowing google review for me and I have not heard from her since.

Phil Cardow   phil@philcardowhypnotherapy.com.au

Chapter 7- Using Self Hypnosis with SP

SP SELF HYPNOSIS

Annamaria La Scala

Self-hypnosis with the Simpson Protocol: a quick and effective process

All hypnosis is self-hypnosis, as it requires active participation by being open to the experience and letting the transformation happen.

Learning to do self-hypnosis with the Simpson Protocol (SP) means acquiring the ability to reach a deep state of hypnosis rapidly and easily and gain trust into the Superconscious to do the work with the best results for our needs and wishes.

The Superconscious, or inner/higher mind, is like a force within us that can help and bring about the changes we want in our life in the most appropriate way for us. Sometimes this happens rapidly, sometimes gradually, but it is always for the best. The key is to stay curious, open-minded and learn to trust the process. This might not be easy at first, but with practice, it becomes easier, quicker and highly effective.

As confidence in the self-hypnosis process strengthens, practitioners can start directly communicating with the Superconscious Mind and make the process interactive, fun and enriching. There is no need to completely clear your mind, no need to let a suggestion "float", no need to spend a long time in a meditative state, unless that's what you are looking for, and the results can be remarkably significant.

You can learn to practice and communicate with the Superconscious with closed or open eyes, sitting still or while moving. It is a versatile process, and it is accessible with or without previous experience in hypnosis. The key is to be open to the process and take the time to build confidence.

The applications are multiple, from everyday concerns to more significant health-related challenges such as self-confidence issues, anxiety, pain management, tinnitus, sleep, chemotherapy side effects and more. It is often a wonder to observe the diverse and creative ways people develop to put self-hypnosis to work, incorporating sometimes different other tools they may have learned previously, like Reiki, Silva method techniques or other approaches.

Real stories can demonstrate the potential and variety of applications. For example, a teacher used self-hypnosis to desensitize himself to clean up after a student threw up in class. He did what was needed without feeling any discomfort, numb to the smell and was very happy with himself.

Another story involves an advanced cancer patient who learned to work with self-hypnosis in a few sessions. Several months later she called to say that she was amazed at how well it worked, she could manage anxiety, sleep, pain issues and chemotherapy side effects.

After a couple of years, she let me know that she was well and still using self-hypnosis.

In short, learning and practicing self-hypnosis with SP is a journey worth taking and an investment for life. It is about curiosity, openness and trust, with the potential to make significant positive changes. The process is accessible, enjoyable and empowers you to create your own transformative path.

How to learn self-hypnosis with SP

There are two ways to learn self-hypnosis with SP: group workshops or private sessions.

Several online or in-person workshops are available worldwide to learn and practice self-hypnosis with SP in 3 to 4 hours.

After a brief introduction, the trainer guides the group into hypnosis following the SP process and installs three keywords. With these words, participants start practicing different ways to go into a state of hypnosis, either guided by the trainer or on their own. This helps them gain confidence and starts integrating the process.

In just a few hours, through group hypnosis, practical exercises and shared experiences, participants gain the tools needed to make positive changes in their life.

For people who prefer private sessions with SP, the three keywords will be given at the first appointment, with a short practice at the end. This might be enough to learn to do self-hypnosis and additional practice can be integrated in later sessions based on individual needs and preferences.

Afterward it is a matter of motivation and personal practice!

Annamaria La Scala Annamaria@lascala-hypnose.ch

174

Chapter 8- Breaking it down.

The Simpson Protocol (S.P.) is infinitely flexible, and infinitely variable process - allowing a Practitioner to deal with any issue or trauma simply and efficiently -and producing great outcomes for the client.

A couple of things:

The Simpson Protocol Process is not simply about Hypnosis.

Ines Simpson always says "Hypnosis isn't the PROCESS. Hypnosis allows you to access THE PROCESS.

The PROCESS being those parts of us that can address the problem, the Trauma, the Disharmony, or a Journey for you.

Simpson Protocol is a process that allows you, as a person, or you, as a Therapist Practitioner, to access those powerful and deep parts of any human being that can, if allowed create massive positive change, on any level, physical, mental, emotional spiritual and more.

Simpson Protocol is not about solving or 'fixing' one issue. It's about going through all the issues necessary to achieve the most Optimum OUTCOME for the Client. Holistic.

S.P. takes the Hypnotist's Judgement out of the process - the whole session is led by the client's Intentions and the Superconscious.

The Hypnotist has no need to be aware of the 'issue' in S.P. The outcome can be achieved without the Hypnotist having any knowledge of their particular problem.

As it is the Client's own Mind that leads the session, any issue of the Client can be addressed.

A simple, flexible, system that uses 'deep' states of Hypnosis and more to access and neutralize the deepest traumas to produce huge positive outcomes simply and quickly.

Who can use Simpson Protocol?

Anyone.

Anyone who wants to either help change in another – or create change in themselves. Anyone. No experience necessary

But as you will see from the entries in this book from people and practitioners all around the world, Simpson Protocol is used by some of the most experienced Hypnosis Practitioners around the world.

A little History

The Protocol was developed, (emerged) over time as Ines Simpson experimented with the process of Hypnosis as a Tool for Change. She wanted to simplify the process to allow her to be more efficient. She wanted to develop a methodology that could take the Hypnotists straight to the heart of any issue, without the Hypnotists having to guess or over analyse. A method that would, in the end take the Hypnotists judgement and subjective opinions and history out of the process. And most important a process that would allow the Client to have their issue resolved without necessarily reliving any trauma and without the necessity of the Hypnotist having any information about their issue.

Over time she found a way to communicate with something she calls the Superconscious Mind - a higher mind perhaps – but something that seems to be able to connect with any and all information needed and has only the client's Higher Needs as its guiding Principle. The subconscious may have the client's self-preservation as its main driving force, this Superconscious Mind seems only to want what is always Optimum and Best for the client.

And this Superconsciousness, allows the Hypnotist to become a guide and facilitator - allowing the Client's own Mind to achieve the optimum result.

So, the Protocol became a method that both simplified and expanded the reach of hypnosis therapy for the Hypnotist Practitioner.

A way for the Hypnotist to always be sure they are dealing with the correct issue at the correct time, and to know that the process, guided by the client's Superconscious only has one desired outcome – the best for the client.

And importantly in cases of abuse or PTSD – there is no need for the client to relate any of the details of the issue or issues to the Hypnotist. The Hypnotist need only know there is an issue, and the client is willing to deal with it, at this time.

It is an Inclusive Holistic System of Hypnosis and Therapy- and while it of course benefits the experienced Hypnotist Practitioner – it is at its core an amazingly simple process, Simple to apply and learn, and all encompassing, taking in every aspect of Modern Hypnosis -so it is also   ideal for the beginner to learn and apply.

Simpson Protocol is an all-encompassing hypnosis system for the beginner or the experienced hypnotist to apply in any niche, practice, or application, where optimum outcomes are desired.

"When I saw Ines Simpson demonstrate the Simpson Protocol - I knew this was what I had been looking for. This is what Hypnosis should be about"

***Stin*-Niels Musche**

What is an SP'er?

Who joins this tribe?

People who use SP, whether for person Self Hypnosis or for a therapy to help others – we call them SP'ers.

And what makes up an SP'er?

Someone who cares deeply about helping themselves and other people. About Balance and Harmony in life. About using the simplest most effective and efficient ways to create this balance and harmony

Is SP just a Spiritual Process?

I think the question is – is SP **also** a Spiritual process?

Ines Simpson says SP deals with the whole being, the physical, the mental, the emotional, and all the rest. And let's call 'all the rest' for sake of simplicity the spiritual bits of a person.

SP is Holistic – that is - it leaves nothing out.

But you talk about 'the soul' and the 'SuperConscious' and 'Bardot' and all kinds of spiritual checks- that makes it very spiritual, doesn't it?

Well SP also checks the DNA, RNA, Cellular Memory, Heart, Telomeres, Gut health, Tissues, Glands, Methylation etc.- all aspects of the physical level – so does that make it just a physical process?

SP covers every aspect of a being.

It's the difference between taking your car to a speedy lube – that will only check oil levels – regardless of the problem – as opposed to a full-service mechanic who checks every aspect of the car- to find the root cause –

whether its in fluids, electrics, transmission, cylinders – anywhere and everywhere. Otherwise, you are not really repairing the car at all, you are just doing patches.

Then you say I get the analogy – but the thing is – transmission and electrics etc. are real things – I don't believe in Soul or Bardot stuff.

Of course, what is or isn't – is not about belief. SP is about the result. Ines Simpson never asks here client to 'believe' anything – just be open to all the positive possibilities that a session may offer.

SP will cover the physical mental, emotional and all the other stuff – which you can call the Spiritual – or just 'all the other stuff.'

Maybe there is no 'other stuff' - but doesn't hurt to check.

What is the SuperConscious?

Ines Simpson always answers this question directly with "I don't know."

The thing about defining something that lives in the universe where there is no language- you define and thus restrict the possibilities of that process. If you say it is 'this' then it will only be 'this' and nothing outside of that. So, in Simpson Protocol we say these things like Soul, Spirit, SuperConscious are code words to represent, but not define.

But if you change the question and ask, 'Whatever it may be, does SuperConscious create the desired outcome in this SP process?"

Then the answer is simple – "Yes always"

A little personal bit – Ines Simpson

So, what, to me, is Simpson Protocol?

A process – an ongoing evolution of Hypnosis for Therapy I took to solve practical problems I encountered with my clients.

A journey of discovery, first with Dr James Esdaile's work and then with Dave Elman and Jerry Kein – all of them moving me forward to become more and more effective and efficient in ways to change any client's negative situations.

These amazing Practitioners taught me to always move forward, experiment – and most importantly -believe -there will always be a way to work through any issue for the client.

For instance -I knew that with the Esdaile State there was profound bypass of the critical factor – but no apparent way to communicate to the client in that state. But being led by Superconscious I found ways to communicate with the Client in the Esdaile state.

I loved Regression work – I used it for all my clients – for everything. It's only later reviewing Jerry Kein's work I even realised that he actually taught things other than Regression!!

As I worked with more and more Clients, I found situations I wasn't able to simply resolve with just Regression or perhaps Chair Therapy etc.

Plus, clients didn't want to tell me their horrific stories – and after a while I didn't want to hear them. But if I didn't know the 'issue', how could I address it?

Again, by experimenting, I found that by allowing (trusting) the SuperConscious and the Client's Higher Mind to do the work, without interference, I found any issue could be worked on, and I didn't need to know the issue.

And even now the Simpson Protocol is not finished. It's not a fixed thing, it's always evolving as I and the other SP Practitioners explored its ever-widening potential.

SP is Holistic (covers everything) and ever open to positive change that produces better outcomes. We're always looking for ways to speed up the process and simplify it.

When I was at the beginning of this process – a session would take up to 3 hours – mostly because I wanted to cover every aspect of the issue, and potential issues, and hadn't learned to allow the Client's Mind and SuperConscious to do the work.

Now a session may take 45 minutes to an hour and covers a multitude of issues in that one session.

And these terms – SuperConscious, Subconscious, Higher Mind and so on – what do they mean?

I find when dealing with 'the mind' we are guessing at words. I say we are using Code Words – words that represent things that cannot really be put into words. Maybe there is no such thing as the Superconscious - maybe it's just a higher ultimate part of us that always seems to respond and produce desired outcome – who knows. It doesn't matter. For me it's the results that matter.

Remember once we start working in levels of the Mind that are not what we call the Conscious Mind – we are dealing in places that have no language – need no language. Places of thoughts, intention, imagination, intuition and more.

Now I have found as SP is taught to more and more Practitioners and they began to use it in their daily practice – 'the field' of SP (as in quantum or morphic field concept) expands, becomes more accepted and accepting – and this allows faster easier sessions and more and deeper reach for SP.

Surrogacy is a snap – with humans or animals.

Fertility issues were cleared sometimes in one session – whether it was male or female issue. Fertility issues after the medical profession had given up – and thousands of dollars had been spent. A simple one or two sessions often create real changes. Again, depending on the client's willingness to allow the process to work.

Birthing where the fetus and mother are deeply connected pre-birth through their own higher minds. Yes, the fetus is 'aware.'

PTSD situations are cleared often in one session. And in some cases, many cases, cancer and other chronic diseases have resolved. (Not in all cases, it's never a guarantee – but in a surprising number). Pain, anxiety, chronic diseases or discomfort can be changed in one session.

SP is very exciting to use and be a part of – to see the outcomes that are possible – in such a simple and flexible system.

Anyone who takes SP – their biggest reaction is to how simple and efficient it is to use. And there is no harm that can be done. And no involved process and guesswork.

INES SIMPSON

I had a hypno student abreaction in class whilst demonstrating an induction on another student.... I moved straight into SP to protect her confidentiality in the group....

Superconscious took over the issue(s) and sorted. She tells me she slept for 24 hours sweated IT out and feels amazing now.

And she had been on dozens of retreats and energy courses to heal previously...

PS I still don't know what the issue is... nor need to.'

Beryl Comar-Hypnotist & Trainer

Limit of Liability and Disclaimer of Warranty

The authors and publishers of this book and the accompanying materials have used their best efforts in preparing this document. The authors and publisher make no representation or warranties with respect to the accuracy, applicability, fitness, or completeness of the contents of this document. They disclaim any warranties (expressed or implied), merchantability, or fitness for any particular purpose. The authors and publisher shall in no event be held liable for any loss or other damages, including but not limited to special, incidental, consequential, or other damages. As always, the advice of a competent legal, tax, accounting or other professional should be sought. The authors and publisher do not warrant the performance, effectiveness or applicability of any sites listed in this book. All links are for information purposes only and are not warranted for content, accuracy or any other implied or explicit purpose.

Copyright © inessimpson.com 2024

Copyright © ebookpress-mge 2024

While attempts have been made to verify information contained in this publication, in view of human errors or changes in technology in the future, neither the authors nor the publisher assumes any responsibility for errors, omissions, interpretations or usage of the subject matter herein. This publication contains the opinions and ideas of its authors and is intended for informational purposes only. The authors and publisher shall in no event be held liable for any loss or other damage incurred from the usage of this publication. Every effort will be made to correct any incorrect or inaccurate information – and corrections can be emailed to mhenderson131@gmail.com

Copyright © inessimpsonhypnosis.com 2016,2024

Copyright © ebookpress-mge 2016,2024

www.ingramcontent.com/pod-product-compliance
Lightning Source LLC
Chambersburg PA
CBHW022206050726
47590CB00002B/661